The Hidden Roots:
A History of Homeopathy
in Northern, Central and
Eastern Europe

Robert Jütte

Impressum

© Institute for the History of Medicine
of the Robert Bosch Foundation

Straussweg 17
70184 Stuttgart
Germany

http://www.igm-bosch.de

Director: Prof. Dr. Robert Jütte

Translation: Margot Saar

Layout: Georg Herrmann

ISBN-10: 3-00-01-8464-3
ISBN-13: 978-3-00-018464-2

Stuttgart 2006

Contents

Introduction 7

Norway 11

Sweden 17

Denmark 23

Finland 31

Estonia 35

Latvia 39

Lithuania 45

Czech Republic 49

Slovakia 63

Hungary 67

Greece 77

Notes 82

Introduction

It was in the year 1840 that two homeopaths, Dr Hože, whose Christian name is unfortunately not known, and Carl Steigentesch from the Moravian town of Brno (today part of the Czech Republic) travelled to Paris together in order to visit their great role model and to take part in the yearly celebrations of the 10th August (anniversary of Hahnemann's doctorate). On their journey and also during their stay in Paris they became acquainted with homeopaths from other countries, among them Georg Heinrich Gottlieb Jahr (1800 – 1875), Johann Joseph Roth (1804 – 1859) and Léon Simon (1798 – 1867), who were in Paris at the time, as well as Benoît Jules Mure (1809 – 1859), who had come from Palermo. There were also a number of other physicians who are not known by name but who are known to have come from Montpellier, Dijon, Bordeaux and Madrid. At this point in time, three years before Hahnemann's death, homeopathy had already grown into a world movement and had become established in South- and North America, in India and in most European countries. Part of the world history of homeopathy has now been written, but there are still white areas on the world map, especially in Europe. This is due, on the one hand, to the lack of interest that traditional medical history has professed towards the history of homeopathy for a long time. On the other hand, it has to do with the fact that in some countries homeopathy has only experienced a renaissance in recent years, while its past development has remained unknown because the tradition had not been fostered for several decades.

We find this lack of knowledge about the roots of homeopathy especially in countries that were under Soviet rule during the 20th century, where homeopathic practice was restricted to a clandestine existence. In a number of Scandinavian countries where homeopathy looks back on a long tradition marginalisation has left large gaps in the collective memory so that today we are faced with the necessity to uncover the alternatives to conventional health care and bring them to light again.

In the introduction to a first attempt at putting together a survey of the worldwide development of homeopathy from its first beginnings to the present time Martin Dinges regrets that due to lack of research some gaps could not be closed.[1] He mentions in particular the chapters on the history of homeopathy in the Czech Republic, Slovakia and Hungary, but also in Russia and the Baltic States. For Scandinavia where he points out Norway and Sweden in particular, he also notes a need for more research.

Ten years have passed since Martin Dinges' book was published. For some countries that are not represented in his World History of Homeopathy (published in German in 1996), like Russia[2], Slovenia[3], Bulgaria[4], Hungary[5], and Iceland[6] we have now reliable contributions most of which are even supported by archive material. Thanks to two surveys Mexico and Malaysia have also appeared on the world map.[7] Some gaps still remained, however, especially concerning countries that only recently joined the European Community (for example the Czech Republic) or also countries that have been members for quite some time, like Greece. In many countries homeopathy is still fighting for official recognition or for the implementation of EU directives on the production of medicines. It certainly is a useful exercise for modern practitioners to look back through the long history of this approach to healing in their country. The same applies to legislators who are, according to EU regulations, obliged to take traditional developments into account.

In the face of this somewhat bleak research situation, the following outline of the history of homeopathy in European countries (which are with the exception of Denmark not included in Martin Dinges' *World History of Homeopathy*) can only be a kind of inventory. There are two other recent publications in English[8], both of them uncritical collections of reports about diverse countries taken from the literature or, in most cases, from the internet. Unlike these, the following compilation tries to put together meticulously pieces of information from printed sources (address directories, journals, brochures, congress reports, medical literature etc) of the 19th and 20th centuries to form a more or less complete picture and supplies all relevant references. Both archive and library of the Liga Medicorum Homeopathica Internationalis (LMHI) which are now kept at the 'Institut für Geschichte der Medizin der Robert Bosch Stiftung' (Institute for the History of Medicine of the Robert Bosch Foundation in Stuttgart) proved to be a rich source of information. Some gaps still remain and it will need extensive and time-consuming research as well as a profound knowledge of the language of the respective country to close them. With this preliminary historical survey the author hopes to awaken an interest in a further pursuance of the subject in the individual countries. The beginning has been made!

Norway

Norway's history is closely linked with that of its two Scandinavian neighbour states Denmark and Sweden. Because of its political support for France during the Napoleonic Wars Denmark had to cede Norway to the King of Sweden in the Peace of Kiel. This surrender did, however, not come into force immediately, with the result that Norway declared its independence and, on 17th May 1814 in Eidsvoll adopted a constitution which, notwithstanding a few minor amendments, has remained valid until today. For the following 91 years Norway was governed in personal union with Sweden. On August 13, 1905 an overwhelming majority of Norwegians voted in a referendum for the dissolution of the union that had been forced onto them. Their chosen king who came from the House of Gluecksburg adopted the Norwegian name Haakon VII (1872-1957). During World War I Norway, along with Denmark and Sweden, remained neutral. King Gustav V of Sweden (1858 – 1950) as well as Haakon VII are said to have been amongst the illustrious patients of the English homeopath Sir John Weir (approx. 1879 – 1971) who took up practice in 1911 at the Royal Homeopathic Hospital. Other famous patients included the British monarchs Edward VII, George V, Edward VIII, George VI and Elizabeth II. Marital connections amongst the highest aristocratic families in Europe might well have played a part in this: the wife of King Haakon VII, Princess Maud[9] (1869 – 1938), was the youngest daughter of King Edward VII. But already during the personal union with Sweden a small number of homeopathic physicians were practising in Norway as the following entries from an address list of 1860 show: district physician Dr Oluf Kaurin (1814 – 1883) and Dr Thorvald Oluf Siqueland (1844 – 1881), both residents of Stavanger.[10] Siqueland emigrated to the United States in 1870. Around 1860, Dr Axel Christian Smith was a practising physician in Telemaken.[11]

A translation of Hahnemann's *Organon* first came out in Norwegian in 1990: *Organon: helbredelseskunstens værktøj*, oversat af Jan Als Johanson Kolding: Thaning og Appel. But already towards the end of the 19th century Norwegian homeopaths had published literature on the subject, for example a certain O. M. Ohm (1848 – 1928) whose handbook *Praktisk Homøopatisk legehåndbok for hvermand* appeared in 1893. Ohm practiced between around 1887 and 1900 in Bergen. Originally he had been a ship's captain and he had sailed around the whole world. At the turn of the century another homeopathic practitioner, a Dr N. W. Anderschou, was registered. He was born in Denmark but moved his practice from Oslo to London and later to Glasgow in the 1920s because of continuing hostility towards him.[12] As early as 1916 the first homeopathic journal *(Homeopatisk Tidskrift)* was published in Trondheim, the Norwegian stronghold of homeopathy. It is not known when this journal ceased to appear. It was resurrected in 1963 under the same title and in the same place. Around 1930 three homeopathic magazines were on the market: *Internacia Homöopatistaro (in Esperanto) and Homøopatiske Forening and Aalesunds Homøopatiske Forening* both published in Bergen.[13] Nowadays, homeopathic associations have their own journals and newsletters, like for example the Norske Homeopaters Landsforsbund which publishes the quarterly *Dynamis* that also includes casuistics.

In 1909, the Norwegian homeopaths met with the naturopaths during a congress in Kristiana. In 1928, Olav

Farstad founded the Bergen Homøopatiske Forening, a homeopathic lay association with several hundred members.[14] The Norges Homøopatforening was founded in 1930 by Einar Larsen and Idar Tindvik, two Trondheim practitioners, together with Ivar Ivarsson Fosse (Hundorp), Edward Liebeck (Tromsø), Henry Braun (Narvik), Mathias Milde (Drammen) and the aforementioned Olav Farstad (Bergen). By 1931 this association had nine members and, in that year, sent a representative to the Liga Medicorum Homeopathica Internationalis (LMHI) conference in Geneva.[15] Two clergymen were the driving force behind this small organisation: Theodor Degen, originally from Sembach in Rhineland Palatinate/ Germany, and Tho Hansen from Iowa/ USA. The association's official language was Esperanto and by 1939 it had been renamed Norske Homøopaters Riksforbund and counted seven members. After World War II the number shrank to five: the Norwegian homeopaths Rolf Auster, a certain Volle, Siegfried Waage, Wdm. Elliassen, Kaare Groven and Ansar Berg. There was still obvious public interest in homeopathy as the founding of the Norsk Homøopatisk Pasientforening (NHP) in 1951 shows. This lay association collected 15,000 signatures and won a court hearing in 1966 with the result that homeopathic medicines were removed from the list of drugs considered illegal under the Law of Quackery and were now freely accessible.[16] In 1997 the NHP counted nationally more than 1600 members.

In 1979 and 1980 two new homeopathic associations were founded: Svenska Homøopaters Riksforbund (initiated by the Arcanum Institute in Gothenburg) and, with the particular support of the Norsk Akademi for Naturmedisin, the

Norske Homøopaters Riksforbund. Already in 1982 the two associations merged into one, the Norske Homøopaters Landsforbund. This new organization did not merely represent one branch of homeopathy; it brought together representatives of classic and complex homeopathy with supporters of iridology, phytotherapy and reflexology.

By 1997 there were already four homeopathic associations (number of members in particular year in brackets): Nordiska Homøopaters Forbund (1997: 7 members), Norges Landsforbund av Homøopraktikere (1993: 135 members), Norske Naturterapeuters Hovedorganisasjon (1994: number of members not known), and the Norske Homøopaters Landsforbund whose predecessor already had had 385 members in 1930.[17] In the meantime, a new union has been formed: the Klassiske Homøopaters Forening, which counted six members in 1999. All these associations are not just open to homeopathic physicians.

Until 1987 there was only one training centre, the Arcanum, which more or less held a monopoly position in Norway. Today there are three private schools, all of them in Oslo: Nordisk Høgskole for Homøopati (NHH); Norske Akademi for Naturmedisin (NAN); Skandinavisk Intstitutt for Klassisk Homøopati (SIKH). The latter offers mainly courses in classic homeopathy while NAN also teaches other naturalistic healing practices. SIKH was founded by Leif Ims and Øyvind Hafsl, both Vithoulkas students. All three schools don't just offer theoretical courses but also practical training in homeopathic clinics. NAN devotes 400 and SIKH 850 hours of the training to homeopathy. SIKH also offers a three-year course for medical doctors, in cooperation with the Royal Homeopathic Hospital in London.

In 1999, a report of the Norwegian Department of Health on alternative healing methods came to the conclusion that homeopathy is an efficient healing practice ('mulig effektiv'). Because of the so-called *Kvakksalverloven* (Law of Quackery) that goes back to the year 1936 homeopaths without medical training are not allowed to treat cancer, thyroid disorders or sexual diseases. Homeopathic doctors are faced with the problem that they are only allowed to use therapies which are efficient and harmless. Homeopathic remedies can be bought over the counter and are prescription-free. Most homeopathic remedies that are not specially prepared by a homeopath are imported, mostly from manufacturers in Sweden, England, Germany and Belgium. Since the foundation of the National Centre for Alternative Medicine in Tromsø homeopathy has not had quite as difficult a standing within the Norwegian state health system as before. Nevertheless, there are still no homeopathic hospitals in Norway, only privately run homeopathic dispensaries. For a survey conducted in 1996,[18] 2019 Norwegian physicians were asked if they would be prepared to work together with homeopaths. It turned out that seven percent had no objections to working together, and a third were at least willing to advise patients to try homeopathy. The majority did not have an opinion because they had no knowledge of the homeopathic method. In general, the physicians who had studied abroad were more open-minded. The doctors who were questioned mentioned in particular anxiety, migraines and hay fever as appropriate indications for a homeopathic treatment.

Sweden

As early as 1826 Göran Wahlenberg (1780 – 1851), a pupil of Linné and professor at the University of Uppsala, lectured on Hahnemann's *Organon*. He was also a well-known botanist, and a flower – the ivy-leafed bell flower (Wahlenbergia hederacea) - was named after him. He himself did not practise homeopathically but continued to lecture on the foundations of homeopathy right up his death.[19]

The first Swedish translation of Hahnemann's main opus appeared in 1835 under the title: *Organon för läkekonst; eller första grunderna till den specifika och homeopatiska sjukbehandlingen/ af Samuel Hahnemann*. The translator was a student of Wahlenberg's, Per Jacob Liedbeck (1802 – 1876) who had started his career as prosector of anatomy in Uppsala and practised homeopathy in Stockholm until his death. He was married to a daughter of the founder of Swedish curative gymnastics, Ling. Arcanum brought out a new Swedish translation of *Organon* in 1980 in Gothenburg. Liedbeck published further writings that dealt with the situation of homeopathy in Sweden and other countries and also with the question of homeopathic therapies (casuistics and remedy testing).[20] The publications of Dr O.F. Axell which appeared from 1910 to 1912 under the title *Homeopatisk Terapi*, with 1500 pages the first Swedish standard work, marked an important step forward. An early paper on homeopathic pharmacology was published by Fredrik Johansson in 1923 in Stockholm.[21] The first materia medica to be translated into Swedish was by Karl Stauffer.[22] Apart from the pharmacologies by Swedish homeopaths others written by foreign authors (like Kent and Vithoulkas) are now available in the Swedish language.[23]

The first homeopathic journal *(Homeopatiska underrättelser för svenska folket)* was short-lived (1855 – 1856). The editor was Dr Liedbeck. Between 1907 and 1912 another journal came out *(Homeopatiens Seger)* first in Örebro, later in Östersund. Dr Hjalman Helledag (1855 – 1922) was the editor who, according to an address list from the year 1911, practised as a homeopathic doctor in Östersund.[24] From 1909 to 1918 the popular journal *Från Homeopatiens värld* was published by Dr Petrie N. Grouleff (1862 – 1931). In 1915, the Svenska föreningen for Vetenskaplig Homeopati, a homeopathic practitioners' association (today a practitioners' and patients' association), brought out its own journal *(Sigyn)*. In 1919, its title was changed to *Homeopatiens Seger* which was not only the name of the journal that had been founded some years previously, but also had the same editor: Dr Helledag. Since 1948 this journal has been published as *Tidskrift för Homeopati*. From 1974 to 1979 *Arcanum: Tidskrift för homeopati* also appeared in Gothenburg.

The first association of homeopaths was the Hahnemannföreningen which had been founded in Gothenburg in 1909 in order to offer free homeopathic treatment for the poor and to start a homeopathic hospital. Three years later the homeopathic doctors in the country joined forces as Svenska Homeopatiska Läkareföreningen. This was initiated by the aforementioned Dr Helledag and Dr Adolf Gröndal (1841 – 1912) from Stockholm. In 1915, the Svenska föreningen for Vetenskaplig Homeopati was founded whose aim it was that homeopathy should achieve parity with allopathy. In 1928, homeopathic practitioners founded the Svenska Homeopaters Riksförbund which today calls itself Svenska Homeopratikers Riksförbund (SHR); there are no medical doctors among its members.

In 1975, Svenska Naturläkarförbundet (SNLF) and Svenska Naturmedicinska Sällskapet (SNS) were founded, both of which adopted the German tradition for alternative healers as their model for membership and training policies. Their members have to follow a fixed study plan of the 1995 Kommittén för Alternativ Medicin and attend a minimum of 40 hours of medical study per week (one year full-time, with main focus on anatomy, physiology and pathology). Among the homeopathic practitioners today are around 136 homeotherapists most of whom are trained in classical homeopathy. In 1985, the Svenska Akademin för Klassisk Homeopati (SAKH) was founded which today has more than 90 members. Apart from that, there is the Hahnemann Collegium (HC) which was founded in 1988. These five associations together counted more than 386 members by the end of the 1990s. In addition, there are the Nordiska Homeopatförbundet (NHF) with around 25 members, Legitimerade Sjuksköterskors Riksförening för Homeopati (LSRH) with 7 members, and Riksförbundet för Klassisk Djurhomeopati (RKD) with around 70 members.

SNLF and SNS belong to the Kommittén för Alternativ Medicin (KAM) which among other things pursues common interests concerning regulations on complimentary medicine in Sweden, Scandinavia, the EU and WHO. KAM also founded a committee for non-conventional medicine, the Nordiska Samarbets-kommittén för icke-konventionell Medicin (NSK) of which five partner associations in Sweden, Finland, Denmark, Norway and Iceland are members. The presidency of this organisation has been held by KAM since its foundation in the year 2000. Together with SAKH, KAM initiated a special council association (Homeopatika Rådet i Sverige) which includes apart from KAM, SAKH, SHR and HC also LSRH and RKD.

In 1872, P. O. Chr. Zetterling from the medical faculty of the university in Uppsala donated a considerable amount of money under the condition that it had to be used for setting up homeopathy courses. In 1912, the faculty which rejected this legacy obtained an expertise both from the medical faculties in Stockholm and Lund which branded homeopathy a false doctrine. Still in 1935, during the LMHI congress in Budapest the Swedish delegate complained about the fact that by then funds of 30,000 krone had accumulated but could not be allocated to their stipulated purpose because the faculty was still in denial.[25] In 1926, the attempt had been made to break the resistance by suggesting to invite Dr Ernst Bastanier (1870 – 1953), a homeopath from Berlin who was known to be scientific and critical, as a lecturer.[26]

Nowadays there are several training centres for homeopathy in Sweden. KAM and its member associations insist on 600 homeopathy hours to gain the qualification of 'authorized homeopath', for practitioners who offer various therapies 250 hours are compulsory. There are several schools that offer homeopathic training, for example Homeopatiform, Arcanum, since 1986 Nordiska Akademi för Klassisk Homeopati (NAKH), International School of Classical Homeopathy, Nordiska Hahnemann Institutet, Materia Medica Roslagen AB, Svenskt Center för klassisk homeopati and NMF-Education (formerly: Naturmedicinska Fackskolan), which has offered a combination of full-time and part-time courses as part of their training programme since 1975. Only few universities, for example the Karolinska Institutet at Uppsala University, offer a small amount of tuition on homeopathy.

The 1913 Medicines Act was in so far a step forward as it declared homeopathic remedies to be on a par with pharmaceutical drugs. Already before World War I there were several homeopathic pharmacies in Sweden, not just in the capital but also in the provinces, for example in Sollefteå, where the German company of Dr Willmar Schwabe (Leipzig) had set up a subsidiary. In the 1970s homeopathic medicines were banned from pharmacies and their sale has not been permitted since. They are exclusively sold in health food stores.

There are now eight homeopathic suppliers in the whole of Sweden, with some of them importing or producing their own medicines as Swedish pharmacies are all in public ownership and are not allowed to sell or produce them. At the end of the 1990s the German company Heel took over the Swedish manufacturer GCG Farmaceutical (today: DCG Nordic AB). Until the beginning of 2006 the Swedish regulatory authority *(Läkemedelsverket)* has registered 478 homeopathic single remedies and 120 homeopathic complex remedies following the so-called simplified procedure that is without information on indication and in dilutions of over 1 to 10,000, which conforms to European homeopathic drug standards.[27]

Although an approved registration procedure for homeopathic remedies does exist the health system does not allow employees like doctors or nurses to apply homeopathy as the Swedish Physicians' Association is not of the opinion that it fulfils modern scientific standards.[28]

Doctors who go against these regulations might experience severe difficulties and are even in danger of losing their licence to practise medicine. Since May 1993 a special license has been granted to the anthroposophic hospital, Vidarkliniken, to sell anthroposophic remedies. The new drug law which is to come into force on May 1st, 2006 maintains this legal possibility for the government to grant a sales license for anthroposophic remedies, if there are special reasons.[29]

In the course of the 20th century the Swedish government made three attempts (1944, 1952 and 1955) at banning homeopathic drugs from being sold, but none of them proved successful. Attempts at preventing lay doctors from practising homeopathy in 1941 and 1950 also failed. Since 1961 the homeopathic approach to healing has been officially recognized but certain restrictions are still in place. In the mid-1930s the prohibition of homeopathy through the Swedish Parliament could be averted thanks to active support from other countries.[30]

Denmark

Already in 1822 the first homeopathic publication came out in Danish. This was a small booklet by Hahnemann translated by Hans Christian Lund (1765 – 1846) under the title *Den homøopathiske Helbredelse-Laeres Aand*.[31] Lund went on to translate several of Hahnemann's writings into Danish, amongst them also his missives on the treatment of cholera *(Sendebrev om Helbredelsen af Cholera og at sikre sig for Smitte ved Sygesengen: tilligemed et oplysende Tillæg af Forfatteren og bekræftende Meddelser af Udgiveren*, Copenhagen 1831) as well as his publication on allopathy *(Alløopathien et Ord til Advarsel for ethvert Slags Syge,* Copenhagen 1831). The first homeopathic compendia and guidebooks for laypersons in Danish were also translated by Hans Christian Lund, for example Carl Georg Christian Hartlaub's introduction to homeopathy titled *Katechismus i Homøopathien eller kort og fattelig Fremstilling af den homøopathiske Lægemaades Grundsætninger for Læger og Ikkelæger* (Copenhagen 1827).

There can be no doubt that, already during Hahnemann's lifetime, a considerable variety of homeopathic writings was available in the Danish language contributing to the promulgation of this approach to healing in Denmark. The bible of homeopathy, Hahnemann's *Organon,* however, was translated into Danish only much later: *Organon: helbredelseskunstens værktøj, oversat af Jan Als Johansen* (Frederiksberg) 1990.[32]

Lund also published the first homeopathic journal in Danish *(Homøopathiken eller Den reformerte Lægekunst, et Ugeblad for Sundheds = og Sandhedsyn-dere)*, of which, however, only a few issues appeared (January to

July 1833). One reason for its early demise, apart from censorship, might well have been lack of time. Only in the second half of the 19th century were new journals initiated: *Homøopathisk Tidskrift* (Aarhus) 1896 – 1902, *Maanedskrift for Homøopathi* (Copenhagen) 1860 – 1897. For some years now the Dansk Selskab for Klassisk Homøopati has been publishing the journal *Hahnegal*.

Lund doubtlessly prepared the ground for homeopathy in Denmark. Originally a ship's doctor, he started practising homeopathically in 1821. Members of the bourgeoisie and upper middle class were the most likely readers of his popular medical translations. It was in these circles that homeopathy was particularly popular as the appeal of Gustav Ludvig Baden (1764 – 1840), a Copenhagen high court judge, to the doctors in 1828 showed, in which he demanded that the new approach to medicine should be tested without prejudice and outcomes and experiences should be reported on. One of the few doctors to take this request seriously was the editor of a medical journal *(Bibliothek for Laeger)*, Dr Carl Otto (1795 – 1879). Initially, he had made no secret of his sceptical attitude but, that notwithstanding, he welcomed Hahnemann's research on the effect of remedies in principle. His own experiments on patients who suffered from different symptoms (chills, stomach cramps, dry cough) confirmed his doubts about the effectiveness of homeopathic remedies and led him to the conclusion that 'it is a real credit to Danish doctors that they never approved of homeopathic remedies'.[33] We know today that Otto used only secondary literature for his therapy tests and that he obtained his homeopathic medicines from a pharmacist who had little expertise in their manufacture.

A few years later, in 1835, a military doctor, Christian Heinrich Hahn (1802 – 1868) wrote about his positive experiences with Hahnemann's medical approach in the same journal. He had to concede, however, that his treatment had not been effective in all cases. He also described his journey to some of the most outstanding homeopaths in Germany. He had visited, amongst others, Hahnemann in Köthen as well as Paul Wolf (1795 – 1857) and Karl Friedrich Trinks (1800 – 1868) in Dresden. Because of numerous contradictions, the article did, however, fail to attract the interest of leading Danish medical circles despite of the fact that the author ultimately emphasized the general correctness of the simile principle. One young physician, Carl Kayser (1811 – 1870), at least, took it on himself to accuse Hahn of methodical negligence. One of the points he made was that placebos had not been used in the drug tests and that the tests had not been performed on healthy people as requested by Hahnemann. The early allusion to placebo-controlled studies is remarkable at a time when these methods were tested for the first time by homeopaths and their critics in Germany.[34]

At the same time, also in 1835, the town physician Holger J. Fangel (1794 - ?), who also practised homeopathically, published his own positive experiences with homeopathy based on 163 case studies from his own practice in Fredericia (Jutland).[35] There were no failures, in all cases the patient was healed, a fact, which probably still did not win over the sceptics. Fangel also pointed out in his paper that homeopathic treatment was cheaper and that it should therefore interest the local authorities. His proof of effectiveness, however, did not remain unchallenged. Several leading Danish physicians accused Fangel of incorrect argumentation and called for controlled clinical tests in accordance with the then up-to-date state of medicine.[36] They referred to the predominantly negative research results from an investigation into homeopathic therapy that had been conducted at the beginning of the 1830s in several European hospitals (Paris, St. Petersburg, Lyon).[37]

It took longer here than in other Nordic countries until homeopaths finally started an association. The Homeopathic Society was only founded in 1854. It had around 100 members in 1884 but by the end of the century membership had shrunk by half. In 1911, it was openly criticized that there was 'a lack of organising spirit' in Denmark.[38] This organising spirit did not surface until 1987 when the Dansk Selskab for Klassisk Homøopati was founded.

Until today homeopathy in Denmark has not managed to enter the medical faculties. Already in 1867 the physician Henrik Lund tried to gain a doctorate at the University of Copenhagen with a dissertation on Arnica as a homeopathic remedy. He failed because the experts were of the opinion that the effects of Arnica described in the thesis were based on unscientific assumptions. This is the reason why homeopaths continue to train abroad or in non-university institutions like the Skolen for Klassisk Homøopati (SKH) which was founded in 1987. None of the courses that this school offers is recognized by the Department of Education. Any practitioner who has not completed a medical training is in danger of being persecuted as a quack. Exceptions are those parts of Schleswig that became Danish after the referendum of 1920. A government decree from 1922 allowed homeopathic lay practitioners in this region as this conformed to German law.

In 1837 there were, after all, four homeopaths for every 71 allopaths in Copenhagen. But the ratio went down in the course of the 19th century. Eight homeopathic physicians were practising in 1884 in the Danish capital, but the number of conventional doctors had by then already risen to 180. The ratio was even worse in the provinces. In Jutland, in 1884, one single practising homeopath competed with 237 allopaths. None of the homeopathic practitioners working in Denmark in the 19th century rose to a leading position, as Anna-Elisabeth Brade has demonstrated. Proponents of Hahnemann's medical method had to be prepared to become complete outsiders. Amongst the best known Danish homeopaths during the first half of the 19th century was Johann Carl Ludwig Pabst (1795-1861) who still practised in Copenhagen around 1860.[39] Others were Hans Thomsen (1802 – 1864), a trained surgeon who excelled in his battle against cholera, and Christian Leontin Lund (1818 – 1875), a son of H. C. Lund.

In 1832, the Danish Chancellery decreed that only qualified doctors should have the right to practise homeopathy. Any other healers were considered illegal under the law of quackery which dates back to 1794 and is still in force today as homeopathy has not been officially recognized yet by the Danish health authorities or by the medical fraternity. In 1854, an illegally practising homeopath and clergyman, Ludvig Daniel Hass (1808 – 1881), at least achieved an amendment of the law which meant that quacks were not punished so severely any more. Hass himself received six sentences for violation of this law which, however, did not keep him from looking for other ways of practising and promoting homeopathy. He would, for example, order remedies for his personal use from abroad, as self medication was not liable to prosecution. He also published a handbook for laymen which was reprinted six times between 1860 and 1881. In the third edition Hass advised his readers to order homeopathic remedies from the Homeopathic Central Pharmacy in Leipzig. According to the 1887 pricelist of this pharmacy one had to pay a fifty *Pfennig* postage for parcels to Denmark that weighed up to five kilos.[40] Only towards the end of the 19th century a few pharmacies in Denmark started to produce and sell homeopathic remedies. An 1894 directory shows two homeopathic pharmacies in Denmark, one of which was in Frederiksberg.[41] Shortly before World War I the company of Dr Schwabe had a dispensary in Copenhagen.[42] In 1931, Schwabe exported homeopathic remedies worth 14,812 Reichsmark to Denmark, nearly as much as to Austria, but this was only a quarter of what was sent to Sweden. Like in other countries, Schwabe's export figures dropped during the 1930s. In 1937, only 7,682 Reichsmark worth of homeopathic remedies were exported from Denmark.[43] Danish homeopaths had lost the right to dispense already at the beginning of the 1880s. They took legal action before the Supreme Court, but without success.

In the 1860s the Homeopathic Society which had been founded in 1854 raised funds to start a homeopathic hospital after the Copenhagen town council had refused permission to integrate a homeopathic department into the municipal hospital. In 1884, a plot of land was purchased for this purpose and in 1913, the hospital was inaugurated. It had 52 beds and offered surgery and physiotherapy as well as electromedical treatment and balneotherapy. Contagious diseases were not treated in this hospital which, only three years after its inauguration, was converted into an ordinary children's hospital. Reverend Hass, the great benefactor of homeopathy, had opened a hospital for chronically ill patients in 1874, which was, however, closed already in 1876 because of structural defects in the building. The director was a veteran of the homeopathic movement in Denmark, Dr Søren Jensen (1811-?). In the 1890s a small homeopathic clinic seems to have existed in Veile. It specialised on stomach problems and its director was Dr Ludvig Hakon Feveile, son of the distinguished Danish homeopath Erik Nisson Feveile (1819 – 1873).[44] In 1888, he published a Danish translation of the homeopathic handbook for laymen by Theophil Bruckner (1821 – 1896), stepping into the editorial footsteps of his father who, in 1867, had written an introduction to Clara Fangel's homeopathic cookbook *(Homøopatisk Kogebog)* and who, until his death, was editor of the homeopathy journal. Another homeopathic hospital *(Homeopatisk Hospital)* with 30 beds opened in Copenhagen (Rosbeckvej 1) in 1925 and still existed at the beginning of the 1930s.[45]

What is special about the situation in Denmark, according to Anna-Elisabeth Brade, is that here, the medical establishment succeeded in excluding homeopathy more successfully than in any other country. One of the reasons why this was possible might be that all the leading conventional physicians as well as the state officials in high government positions had studied at the same university and had the same social background. This alleviated the growth of a network of relationships and favoured the tendencies for monopolization within the Danish medical fraternity more than anywhere else. What played also a part was the fact that, already around the middle of the 19th century, hydropathy was competing with homeopathy. The following slightly ironic remark was found in the British Journal of Homeopathy in 1855: 'If homeopathy has not made that progress in Denmark which we might have expected from the great intelligence of the people, hydropathy at least can boast a very large number of partisans.'[46]

Veterinary homeopathy was for a long time equally frowned upon in Denmark. The *International Directory* of 1911 boasts only one single vet, but contains the following notice: 'There are others who ask not to be known as homeopaths as there is no certain organization.'[47] Nevertheless, veterinary homeopathy was apparently very popular amongst Danish farmers at the time.

Finland

The history of homeopathy in Finland is, in its early stages, closely linked with that of the Tsardom.[48] In 1809, Sweden had to cede its former province Finland to Russia. Since that time Finland was, as a grand duchy, in a personal union with the Russian crown. It could, however, retain for a short time Swedish private law, its own political organs and currency. In the Finnish revolution of 1917 it separated from the Russian empire. In 1919, Finland adopted a republican constitution which, after a short interplay involving a monarch, came into force.

Already shortly before the German-French war the governor-general of Finland, Count Nikolai Adlerberg (1819 – 1892), invited one of the most renowned German homeopaths, Dr Eduard von Grauvogl (1811 – 1877) to come and introduce homeopathy in Helsinki.[49] Grauvogl accepted the invitation in November 1871, under the condition that he could bring a reliable pharmacist with him, a wish he was granted. Grauvogl described the resistance he was faced with in a letter that he wrote a few years later to a Russian physician. Grauvogl's lectures, to which no medical students but only qualified doctors were admitted, were also attended by two high-ranking military physicians and by the head of the medical faculty of the university and a general practitioner. Only the two military physicians remained faithful to him. The Tsar had even given orders to reserve two sickrooms in the Helsinki military hospital for Grauvogl, where he could treat his patients exclusively homeopathically. Grauvogl also operated a successful private practice which attracted patients from as far away as St. Petersburg. But it was not long before Grauvogl complained about intrigues from his opponents, among them the head of the health department who was said to be hostile towards homeopathy. Grauvogl was unhappy about the fact that only chronically ill patients were transferred to his homeopathic ward in the military hospital because it meant that his success rate deteriorated. He also found that Count Adlerberg did not keep his promises. For one thing, he had been promised a newly built pavilion for homeopathic treatment, a project which kept on being postponed. When his benefactor fell seriously ill while they were together on an inspection journey through the country, Grauvogl had to devote himself entirely to his important patient. During all that time he was fully conscious of the consequences he would have to face in case his homeopathic treatment should prove unsuccessful. As it happened, the governor-general did recover his health and the Tsar bestowed the second class Order of St. Anne on Grauvogl. Nevertheless, our pioneer of homeopathy in Finland was not prepared to put up with any more hostilities. He returned to his homeland and, in 1873, finally settled down in Munich.

That this was not the end of homeopathy in Finland is shown by a critical essay written by A. Pfaler on the subject of quackery which was published in a Finnish journal in 1888.[50] An article that was printed a few decades later in the same journal also speaks about the quacks and the tricks they were up to in Finland.[51] At the same time it informs us that homeopathy was particularly widespread in the Swedish speaking western part of the country, while in other parts only a small number of travelling homeopaths was practising.

It was only in the 1980s that homeopathy became important in Finland.[52] In 1984, the first efforts were made towards forming a homeopathic association. They were initiated by homeopathic physicians who had studied in Sweden. At the beginning of the 1990s there were already two homeopathic professional societies in Finland: Suomen Homeopaatitry, since 1991 ECCH member, and Suomen Klassiset Homeopaatitry. Their members were mostly recruited from the graduates of the Finnish School of Classical Homeopathy. The two associations whose aim it was to promote classical homeopathy merged into one in 1994. The graduates of the Luontaislääkinnän edistämiskeskus also formed a union called Pohjoismainen Homeopaattiyhdistysry (The Nordic Homeopaths). This society counted around 50 members at the end of the 1990s while the bigger association, Suomen Homeopaatitry had more than 400 members, among them 160 practising homeopaths.

In Finland, homeopaths train in special institutions: Homeopatia Institute, the Finnish School of Classical Homeopathy in Helsinki, and Luontaislääkinnän edistämiskeskus (Centre promoting naturopathic medicine) near the city of Tampere. The training programme includes a medical foundation course of 600 hours which are partly taught in cooperation with the medical school of the University of Helsinki.

Finland has only had a homeopathic journal of its own since 1992: *Homeopatia* which is published by the Finnish Homeopaths' Association. Introductions to homeopathy in Finnish have only been available since the 1970s: H. Åberg, *Homeopatia*. Kirjasepot, Pieksämäki 1977; A. Voegeli, *Homeopaattisen hoidon aakkoset*.

WSOY, Porvoo 1988 (translated from the German); G. Vithoulkas, *Homeopatia. Tulevaisuuden lääketiede.* WSOY. Juva 1990; C.D.O. Pellas, *Homeopatian aakkoset. Homeopatiens ABC*, Nekapaino. Tampere 1990; D. M: Gemmel, *Homeopaattinen kotihoito. Homeopaattien Farmasia* RL Oy. Hameenlinna 1991. In the early stages, people got by with Russian text books, as one can see from Finnish library catalogues, and in the first half of the 20th century they probably read the relevant literature in Swedish.

Today, homeopathy is still not officially recognized in Finland and the name 'homeopath' is not legally protected either. Homeopathic remedies, however, have to be registered in Finland before they can be sold because registrations from other EU countries are not accepted.

Estonia

Estonia as we know it today consists of the former Baltic province of Estonia (which until 1918 belonged to the Russian Empire) and the Northern part of Livonia which also includes the island Saaremaa. During the October Revolution of 1918 Estonia gained independence. The Soviet Union put massive pressure onto the Baltic States and annexed them in 1940 (Estonian Socialist Soviet Republic), having sent in Russian troops already earlier on. From 1941 to 1944 the country was occupied by the Germans. After renewed occupation through the Red Army in the autumn of 1944, the country was re-annexed by the Soviet Union following the Yalta Conference. In August 1991, after several years of negotiations, Estonia finally regained its independence.

Similarly to the political history, the history of homeopathy in Estonia is closely connected with the development and the restrictions it experienced in the Tsardom.

According to the Ukase of 26th September 1833 the practice of homeopathy was officially permitted in the Tsardom, but only for medical school graduates. In addition, homeopathic pharmacies were expressly permitted in the provinces. In exceptional cases homeopathic physicians were even granted permission to have their own dispensary. Hahnemann's doctrine had found supporters in Estonia already some years before. The centre of this movement was Tartu where Dr Ludwig Reinhold von Stegemann (1795 – 1849) was active at the beginning of the 1820s. He had been appointed Privy Councillor by the Tsar because of his medical achievements. In 1825, he wrote from Tartu to Dr Johann Ernst Stapf (1788 – 1860), editor of the *Archiv für die homöopathische Heilkunst* (Homeopathy Archives), that he 'was not exactly unhappy as a practitioner of homeopathy' and he described two of his recent cases where the patients had been cured. His letter ends with the words: 'It shall be an honour and joy to me to actively propagate this naturalistic healing method in Russia and Livonia.'[53] Stegemann had already healed the wife of a certain Christoph Kaule in Riga in 1823 who consequently became a fervent sponsor of homeopathy.[54] After a few interim positions Stegemann practised again in Tartu at the beginning of the 1830s. But his success led Gottlieb Franz Immanuel Sahmen, who was professor for pharmacology at the University of Tartu from 1826 to 1828, to pen a critical paper in which he did not actually generally reject homeopathy as inefficient but refused the exclusiveness that Hahnemann and others claimed for their healing approach. He described homeopathic experiments that he himself had conducted and had not found satisfactory.[55]

There can be no doubt that, already in the 1820s, homeopathy had found supporters as well as opponents in the area that is now Estonia. The sources do not reveal anything more about its further propagation. A job advertisement published in a German specialist journal in 1855 gives the impression that homeopathy must have continued to be quite popular in Estonia: in Kertel an 'experienced homeopathic physician'[56] was needed by several landowners who were prepared to offer a salary of 600 taler as well as a practice with 16 to 20 beds in a hospital. Around 1850 a homeopathic doctor named Carl Abraham Hunnius (†1851) lived in Haapsalu. He was originally from Reval and had written his doctoral dissertation at the University of Tartu on 'anthrax carbuncles'.[57] From 1830 onwards he had practised as a homeopath. Another practitioner was a certain Dr Heinrich who lived in Tallinn (Reval) in the 1840s. He complained, in 1844, in the *Allgemeine Homöopathische Zeitung* (German homeopathic journal) about Dr Buchner's judgment on homeopathy in Russia.[58] In Tartu, the aforementioned Dr Stegemann was succeeded by the physician Dr von Holst.[59] Most certainly this was Johannes von Holst who had gained a doctorate in 1848 in Tartu with a dissertation about the muscle structure.[60] In Pärnu there were two homeopathic physicians in the second half of the 19th century: Dr Carl Adolph Knorre (†1870) who defended his dissertation in Tartu in 1822, and Dr Friedrich Gottlieb Landesen, who ran his medical practice for nearly 50 years as a homeopath before he retired. He, like his colleague, held a medical doctorate from the University of Tartu.[61] Between 1802 and 1898 the official language of the University of Tartu was German. Many of the professors teaching there were of German origin, too. Especially civil servants and physicians for the entire Tsardom were trained at this academic institution.

The fact that some of the doctors mentioned above were writing for German-language journals shows that in Estonia fundamental homeopathic literature was read in this language. Since 1835 a Russian translation of the *Organon* had also been available.[62] One year previously Hartlaub's short description of the homeopathic healing method had been published in Moscow. From the mid-1830s onwards the number of Russian translations of homeopathic publications increased considerably as is shown by Bojanus' compilation.[63]

There seems to have been a homeopathic pharmacy in Tallinn at the beginning of the 20th century. As in the Soviet Union, homeopathy in Estonia seems to have lost more and more ground after the First World War. No Estonian representatives were present on the LHMI conferences. One of the most famous Estonian homeopaths, Dr Alexander Rosendorff (1871 – 1963) had to leave the country in 1942. He had studied medicine in Tartu and was introduced to naturopathy by Dr Heinrich Lahmann in Dresden. He also became acquainted with electrohomeopathy when he met Cesare Mattei (1809 – 1896). The sign which he had installed in 1920 outside his practice in Reval, Waldstraße, however, said: 'homeopath'. This practice in which he obviously applied a great variety of alternative therapies was so successful that, according to a contemporary,[64] that his patients happily endured long waiting times. Under Soviet rule homeopaths had a difficult life as their healing methods did not conform to the Pavlov-influenced traditional medical approach that was popular with party members.[65] But at about the same time as perestroika spread in the Soviet Union homeopathy in Estonia experienced a revival: At the beginning of the 1990s a few Russian physicians began to practise homeopathically. The first congress took place in 1996.[66] In 1997, the Estonian Society of Homeopathy was founded which counted more than 50 members at the dawn of the 21st century. Some of them also belonged to the LMHI. In 1999 this association was granted, by the Estonian authorities, the privilege to issue tax deductible donation receipts. In 2001 it came to a split in this organisation, probably due to the wide ranging political interests of its members.[67]

In 2000, the first training courses of the Belgian-Russian Classical Homeopathy School began. German pharmaceutical companies are now offering introductory courses. Today, literature on homeopathy is also available in the Estonian language.

Latvia

Similar to other Baltic States Latvia's history shows a series of fractures which also affected the history of homeopathy in these parts of Europe. The Treaty of Nystad in 1721 declared Livonia and Estonia to be Russian provinces. With the third Partition of Poland in 1795 Kurland and Polish Livonia (Lettgallen) became Russian. Together with Estonia, they formed the Baltic 'gouvernements' that enjoyed special status. With the end of the First World War German occupation also ended and the declaration of independence was pronounced on 18th November 1918. In October 1939 the Soviet Union forced an assistance and military base agreement on Latvia. Due to an additional protocol to the Hitler-Stalin-Pact the country fell under Soviet influence and had to consent to Soviet troops being stationed here. The occupation began on 17th June 1940 and was followed soon after by the occupation through German troops during World War II. In the autumn of 1944 the country was almost entirely re-conquered by the Red Army and, after the war, it was annexed by the Soviet Union as the Latvian SSR. On 4th May 1990, Latvia declared independence. The independence of Latvia, Lithuania and Estonia was recognized by Russia on 21st August 1991.

Already during Hahnemann's lifetime the first publications on homeopathy appeared in Riga. In 1838, Dr Carl Ernst Brutzer (1794 – 1877) published a German opus with the title *Versuch einer theoretischen Begründung des Princips der Homöopathie, nebst einigen Folge- und Nebensätzen für Ärzte*. (Attempt at a Scientific Foundation of the Homeopathic Principle).[68] It was intended as a guidebook cum materia medica. Already in 1833, Brutzer had asked the society of physicians of which he was a member: 'Should it be possible for a conscientious physician of our times to leave homeopathy unexamined?' and he answered the question himself by describing some cases from his homeopathic practice. He also offered a prize of 100 ducats for an unbiased research paper on homeopathic case studies.[69] Brutzer continued to practise in Riga to a very high age and celebrated his golden jubilee as a doctor in 1872. Only around the turn of the 20th century the first Latvian translations of homeopathic works came out, among them a book for laypersons with excerpts from different popular guidebooks (Hering, Lutze etc.). It had been translated by a certain J. Berzinsh.[70] Another author of lay publications was a man called Lapmezhs. The most productive translator at the time was M. Shimminsh, who, financially supported by the owner of the homeopathic pharmacy in Riga, translated several German books into Latvian. There were, however, not only translations from the German but also from the Russian language, for example a lecture that Dr Lev Brazol (1854 – 1927) gave during the All Russian Homeopathic Congress in St Petersburg in 1913 with the title *Modern Homeopathy*.

One standard work of homeopathy, Willmar Schwabe's *Pharmacopea homeopathica polyglotta* (1880) had for a long time only been available in the German language, but was finally translated into Russian in 1957. After World War II it became more difficult to publish homeopathic literature. Dr G. Kundzina, for example, translated a book by Herwig Storch, *Homöopathische Arzneimittel für die Praxis* (Remedies for the Homeopathic Practice, 1956) into Latvian, but the translation remained unpublished. Only towards the end of the 1990s Russian translations of

Kent's and Hering's Materia Medica found their way into Latvian medical libraries.[71]

Homeopathic physicians who practised in Latvia in the 19th and early 20th century were often corresponding members of the St. Petersburg homeopathic societies or other foreign homeopathic associations.[72] Only when Latvia regained independence, in 1991, the Latvian Homeopathic Association (LHA) was founded, but it was not officially registered until 1995. After that it received, from the Latvian Medical Association, the right to add the title 'Homeopathy' to that of medical doctors, who have to account for five years of practical experience before they can assume that title, though. The first president of this association was Dr B. Limba. She also belonged to the Moscow Homeopathic Association. Since 1998 LHA is a member of the Liga Medicorum Homeopathica Internationalis. In 2001, 53 medical doctors were members of the LMHI in Latvia.[73]

A lay association seems to have existed already at the beginning of the 20th century. Its president was the aforementioned translator M. Shimminsh.

Still in the year 1999 the association of homeopathic doctors in Latvia complained about the absence of a Latvian journal, a situation which has not changed up to now.

One of the first tasks of the Homeopathic Doctors' Association that was founded in 1991 was the organisation of training courses. Although there was some expertise in the country most doctors who were interested in homeopathy learned about it abroad, in particular in the courses that George Vithoulkas hosted at his centre in Greece. In 2000, the Baltic Centre of Classical Homeopathy was founded. By the year 2000, 69 doctors had successfully graduated from the seminars that the LHA has offered since 1991. Apart from Riga, homeopaths are still mostly trained in homeopathic training centres that had been important before the country became independent, i.e. in Kiev and Moscow. In the 1920s Latvian doctors also attended vocational training courses in the Homeopathic Hospital in Stuttgart/Germany.[74]

Since Hahnemann's lifetime until today there has been an ongoing tradition of homeopathic physicians in Latvia. In the 1840s physicians like Dr Lembke in Riga even treated cholera patients as suggested by Hahnemann: with camphor.[75] A directory of homeopathic doctors lists under 'Riga' for the year 1860 the doctors Brutzer and Lembke both of whom have been mentioned here already, and also Dr Brauser (große Schloßstraße), Dr Hencke (Scheunenstraße) and Dr Riedel (kleine Schmiedstraße).[76] It is impossible to establish if there were any homeopathic practitioners among the veterinary doctors listed in the 1862 medical directory for Riga.[77] Around 1880, Dr Heinrichsen and Dr Schreckenfels practised homeopathically in Riga.[78] Dr Riegel was also still active there at that time. There was a homeopathic physician in Jelgava (Mitau) in the second half of the 19th century too: Dr Theodor Meyer.[79] Around the year 1894 Dr Eduard von Erdberg who had studied in Petersburg practised in Riga, as well as Dr Theodor Rollseun, who had previously worked in Tartu.[80] Shortly before World War I an international address directory lists next to Dr Rollse[u]n also a certain Dr Zelenkow.[81] Amongst the most important though not 'classical' homeopaths in Riga at the beginning of the 20th century was Dr Feliks Lukin (1875 – 1934) who was particularly interested in electrohomeopathy as well as Ayurvedic and Tibetan medicine. His son, Dr Harald Lukin (1906 – 1991) also practised homeopathically in Latvia and is said to have treated between 50 and 80 patients per day, some of them coming from as far away as Moscow. At the beginning of the 1930s there were 16 homeopathic physicians in Riga alone. One of them was Dr E. Epplee who had worked in Moscow before.[82] Immediately after the Second World War the following homeopathic doctors practised, among others, in Latvia, some of them under very adverse circumstances: Dr Martene, Dr Leja, Dr Kruminsh, Dr Vulfins, Dr Paukshene, Dr Burstein, Dr Asinas and Dr Ivochkins. Of these only the name of Dr Burstein appears again in the (albeit incomplete) 1966 *World Directory of Homeopathic Physicians*.

Already in 1833 a homeopathic pharmacy opened in Riga which belonged to the Riga Chemo-Pharmaceutical Society in whose ownership it remained until 1848. It was the first of its kind in the Tsardom. The number of prescriptions that were issued there grew from 2,983 in 1834 to 23,420 in the year 1874.[83] Around 1860 this pharmacy belonged to four allopathic chemists.[84] In 1898, another homeopathic pharmacy opened. The *International Homoeopathic Directory* of 1911/12 mentions, apart from the oldest pharmacy, that of Johannes Stein in Wallstraße as a general agency of the company Willmar Schwabe for all of Russia. In 1939, there were already five homeopathic pharmacies in Latvia, four in Riga and one in Liepāja. After World War II only the pharmacy with the longest tradition remained and continued to supply the entire country with homeopathic remedies. Since 1940 it had been owned by Egon Dilbeck who remained responsible for it even after its nationalisation. In 1950, Mrs Mirdza Ozolina took over its management. She continued to run it until the year 2000 and has since supported it on an honorary basis. Until 1991 this central pharmacy supplied all other Baltic states as well as Belarus with homeopathic remedies.

Latvia's first homeopathic polyclinic was founded in Riga in 1965. This was an initiative of Mrs Mirzda Ozolina, the director of the central homeopathic pharmacy, an outpost of the Moscow Homeopathic Hospital which, however, was closed down again after only a few months due to pressure from the party leaders. A second attempt in 1966 proved more successful. The homeopathy department was part of polyclinic number 5 in Riga. Eighteen homeopathic physicians are said to have been working there already in 1970. The endeavour of Boris Petrovsky (1908 – 2004), who was Russian health minister at the time, to close down this department was futile, because the effectiveness of the treatment could be proved.[85] Until today the homeopathic method only plays a marginal role in Latvia's hospitals.

Lithuania

Lithuania became a Russian province after the third "Partition of Poland" (1795). In 1812, Napoleon's revolutionary army occupied the Baltic States. The Lithuanians welcomed the French troops as their liberators. After the retreat of the French, Tsar Nicholas I began to massively russify Lithuania. After World War I, the Treaty of Versailles granted Lithuania de jure independence on 28th June 1919. The Soviet Union accepted Lithuanian independence in the Moscow Peace Treaty of 1920. For a short time Lithuania was a parliamentary democracy but soon, in 1926, became an authoritatively governed country. At the end of March 1939, under pressure from Hitler, Lithuania had to cede the Memel District (Memelland) to Germany. After the German attack on Poland in September 1939 the Red Army entered the Baltic States and East Poland under the Hitler-Stalin-Pact. The formal Russian annexation of Lithuania as the Lithuanian SSR followed in July 1940. With the beginning of the Russia Campaign the German Wehrmacht (Armed Forces) occupied Lithuania. In 1944 it was re-conquered by the Red Army. The russification of Lithuania was further increased after World War II and led to violent acts of resistance. In the mid-1980s the Lithuanian independence movement emerged. In March 1990 the parliamentary chairman Vytautas Landsbergis declared Lithuania's independence. In 1993 the country became a member of the Council of Europe.

As with the other Baltic States that regained their independence in 1990 Lithuania's history of homeopathy is closely linked to that of Russia.

During the second half of the 19th century Polish as well as Russian translations of homeopathic standard works were widely read in Lithuania. In 1850, Dr Piletzky published a Polish version of Constantin Hering's *Homöopathischer Hausarzt* (Homeopathic Family Doctor) in Kaunas (Kovno). The Polish translation *(Dyetetyka homoeopatyczna)* of a paper by the German-Hungarian homeopathic physician Franz Hausmann (1811 – 1876) was published in Vilnius in 1858.[86] The first Lithuanian book on homeopathy came out in 1907.[87]

It was only at the beginning of the 1990s that homeopaths in Kaunas founded their own association. Since 2002 the members of the Lithuanian Homeopathic Doctors' Association have been LMHI members. During the first decade following the declaration of independence there were over one hundred accredited homeopaths in Lithuania. Today there are several homeopathic organisations in Lithuania: The Centre of Homeopathic Medicine, The Association of Lithuanian Homeopaths, The League of Medicinal Homeopathy, the Association of Homotoxicology and Antihomotoxic Therapy.[88]

During the first half of the 19th century, a student of Hahnemann's, Dr Julius Niklewicz (1802 – 1841) practised in Lithuania. He had studied medicine in Vienna and came originally from Lviv (Lemberg). In 1831, he arrived in Kaunas where he began to practise homeopathically. Around 1835, he was the family physician of a landowner named Johann von Gruzewski in Kelmé. His reputation as a successful homeopath spread far beyond the borders of the little town which was situated about 15 miles from Šiauliai, now an international airport. He died already in 1841 of consumption.[89] At the beginning of the 1870s a certain Dr von Jawlowski practised in Kaunas. He was also known to be a follower of nudism and his homeopathic practice was influenced by the writings of Franz Hartmann (1796 – 1853).[90] In Kaunas an aristocratic lay healer named Kuschelewsky practised around 1880.[91] In Vilnius the doctors Theuillé and Dr Wenblewsky had their practices.[92] Whether the latter is identical with the Dr Wroblewsky who is listed in the homeopathic directory of 1860 cannot be established.[93] In 1894, a directory lists three homeopathic physicians for Riga: Dr Aschkouroff, Dr Xavier Pawlowitsch and Dr Constantin Franzovitsch Schvezkovsky (Schweykovsky).[94] Apart from the last mentioned homeopathic doctor two others, Dr Dunkel and Dr P. Frohwein (Frovein)[95] practised in Vilnius in 1911. Not far from what is now the Lithuanian border, in Sovetsk (until 1946: Tilsit), homeopathy was also widespread around 1850. In the town itself a certain Dr Aszpodin practised at the beginning of the 1870s. Among the rural population the lay healers who were followers of Arthur Lutze's were apparently very popular.[96] In Shvekshny (Sveksna) two homeopathic physicians are mentioned in the year 1894: Dr Dlugoborsky and Ferdinand Matwievitsch.[97]

The first homeopathic pharmacy was set up in Vilnius in 1864. Twenty years later in Kaunas a first pharmacy opened (proprietor: M. M. Klimoritsch) followed by a second one soon after.[98] In Šiauliai, the homeopathic pharmacy Salomon Slavit had opened in 1884 and was open during the early 1890s.[99] The directory of 1894 lists 'Pharmacie L. J. Seidler' in Vilnius which according to the entry was set up in 1857.[100] A later directory lists the 'Pharmacy of the Society of Homeopathy' in the Georgieffski prospectus.[101] Between 1920 and 1984 there was a homeopathic pharmacy in Kaunas (Matulaitis &

Mačius). Since 1992 there has been a homeopathic dispensary here again which continues the earlier tradition. In Kelmé there was also a homeopathic pharmacy towards the end of the 19th century. Its proprietor was M. Sch. Lipschütz.[102]

With regard to the dispensary right the same regulations applied in the 20th century as before in the Tsardom. Nowadays every physician is allowed to prescribe homeopathic medicines in Lithuania, but in order to specialise he or she has to complete additional studies at Kaunas Medical University or at Vilnius University. They are, however, no substitute for the introductory courses in homeopathy that are offered by the Lithuanian homeopathic societies.

Czech Republic

Until 1992 the Czech Republic was, together with Slovakia, part of a state which was officially called *Czechoslovak Republic* from 1918 to 1939, and after World War II *Czechoslovak Socialist Republic* or *Czech and Slovak Federative Republic*. The former Czechoslovakia consisted of the regions Bohemia, Moravia, Czech Silesia (the former Austrian Silesia with the then Prussian region around Hlučín but without an area east of Cieszyn (Teschen; which became Polish), Slovakia and Sub-Carpathian Rus (Podkarpatskà Rus). Up to the end of World War I most of these territories had been part of the Austrian-Hungarian Monarchy. For this reason the history of homeopathy in what is now known as the Czech Republic is closely related to that of Austria. It is a known fact that homeopathic medicine was prohibited under Metternich in 1819 due to the old medical legislation which threatened penalties to doctors who produced their own remedies.[103] Although Emperor Ferdinand I abolished his predecessor's law in 1837, it was only on 9th December 1846 that a Court Chancery decree granted homeopathy equal status with allopathy in all territories, including Bohemia and Moravia.[104]

An early and comprehensive critique of Hahnemann's *Organon* interestingly appeared in Prague in 1819. Its author was the medical professor Ignaz Rudolph Bischoff (1784 – 1850). His polemics begin with a snide remark about the 'unbelievable stir that had been caused by the homeopathic healing method among wide parts of the public'.[105] There can be no doubt that Hahnemann's doctrine and his written works were known in Bohemia which was to a certain extent German speaking at the time, and also in Moravia, although his main opus was translated into the Czech language only in 1993.[106]

In Prague, the capital of Bohemia, the first handbooks and introductions to homeopathy came out already in the first half of the 19th century but they were written in German. One of the best known authors of these fundamental writings was without doubt Elias Altschul (1797 – 1865): *Der homöopathische Zahnarzt*, 1841 (The Homeopathic Dentist); *Lehrbuch der physiologischen Pharmacodynamik*, 1853 (Textbook of Physiological Pharmacodynamics); *Taschenwörterbuch der Kinder-Krankheiten und ihre homöopathische Behandlung: mit steter Angabe der neuern einfachen Heilmittel der physiologischen Schule für Ärzte und Wundärzte*, 1863 (Pocket Dictionary of Children's Diseases and Their Homeopathic Treatment, including the newest simple remedies of the physiological school for physicians and surgeons). His *Klinisch-homöopathisches Taschenwörterbuch für das Haus und die Reise*, 1861 (Clinical Homeopathic Pocket Dictionary for Home and Abroad) as well as his *Real Lexicon für homöopathische Arzneimittellehre, Therapie und Arzneibereitungskunde*, 1864 (Encyclopaedia for Homeopathic Medicines, Therapy and Remedy Preparation) were published in a different place (Sondershausen), where also the works of other important Czech pioneers of homeopathy came out. Among them was also the two-volumed *Die homöopathische Therapie auf Grundlage der physiologischen Schule: ein praktisches Handbuch für Ärzte, welche die homöopathische Heilkunde kennenlernen und am Krankenbette versuchen wollen*, 1865 – 1869, by Jacob Kafka (1809 – 1893) (Physiologically Based Homeopathic Therapy: a practical guide for physicians willing to get to know and practise homeopathic medicine). Czech translations of the most important materia medica editions which are still in use today, for example by James Tyler Kent, became available only much later, in the 1990s, when there was a growing demand for Czech literature on homeopathy.[107]

Already in the first half of the 19th century there were homeopathic journals in German to which practising Bohemian and Moravian homeopaths were contributing, for example the *Austrian Journal for Homeopathy* (1844 – 1849) or the *Journal of the Homeopathic Doctors' Association in Austria* (1862 – 1863). In Prague appeared, between 1853 and 1864, a *Monthly Journal for Theory and Practice of Homeopathy* (from 1855: *Prague Medical Monthly Journal for Homeopathy, Balneotherapy and Hydropathy*). Elias Altschul, of whom we have already heard, copy-edited this journal until his death. When the journal ceased to appear in 1865, homeopathic doctors in Bohemia and Moravia mostly read the General Homeopathic Journal *(Allgemeine Homöopathische Zeitung)*, which was copy-edited from 1872 to 1876 by the aforementioned Dr Jacob Kafka. Between the wars another journal became available: *Hippokrates,* which was published from 1928 to 1978 in Stuttgart/Germany.[108] A Czech journal only came out in the 1990s: *Homeopatická akademie* (Classical Homeopathy) has been published regularly since 1996. The publisher is Alternativa-Verlag which specialises in translations of homeopathic literature into the Czech language. The Czech Medical Homeopathic Society (CLHS) has been publishing for some years now the quarterly newsletter *Homeopaticke listy* (Homeopathic Letters).

The homeopaths who were practising in the 19th century in Bohemia and Moravia were usually members of the Austrian Homeopathic Doctors' Association, which had been founded in 1846 and already had 60 members by 1848. In 1857, an association meeting discussed a question that had been brought up by Dr Altschul, namely, whether the founding of local associations was advisable especially in the countries that were part of the Habsburg Empire.[109] But this does not seem to have happened as the relevant literature does not mention any new foundations, certainly not in Bohemia or Moravia.[110] One of the pioneers of homeopathy in Moravia, for example, the surgeon Anton Fischer (1792 – 1864), who knew Hahnemann personally and who had become famous as a successful healer far beyond his own town (Brno), was a corresponding member of the German Central Association of Homeopathic Physicians in Leipzig and of the corresponding Austrian Association in Vienna. A preliminary directory of the Austrian Homeopathic Doctors' Association from 1857 lists five physicians and surgeons alone from Bohemia and Moravia. With homeopathy having been taboo during the time of the Socialist Republic, only now, at the beginning of the 1990s, an association of homeopathic doctors came about. The Česká lekarska homeopatická spolecnost (Czech Medical Homeopathic Society) was founded in 1990 and recognized by the Czech Association of Physicians in 1993. In the year 2001, this organization had 230 members. Apart from that there is now also the Česká Homeopatická spolecnost (Czech Homeopathic Association, HS) in Prague and the Česká komora klasické homeopatie (Czech Chamber of Classical Homeopathy, KKH) in Brno (Brünn).[111]

The first homeopathic doctor in Bohemia was the Austrian Dr Matthias Marenzeller (1765 – 1854).[112] He became surgeon major at the Prague 'House of Invalids' in 1816. In 1815, he had begun to study homeopathy. He was the first physician in Austria to openly devote himself to homeopathy. Marenzeller was not in the least disconcerted by the fact that homeopathy became prohibited in 1819 in the Austrian 'Erbländer' (hereditary lands). He was, after all, personal physician to Archduke Johann of Austria. In 1829, he moved to Vienna where, until his death, he kept a flourishing practice. Only a few years later, the aristocrat Friedrich Edmund Peithner Ritter von Lichtenfels (1795 – 1857), who, in 1823, lived close to Prague with his family and who later rose to the post of personal physician to the governing prince of Liechtenstein, discovered his interest in Hahnemann's doctrine. He started a homeopathic practice which he continued later, after his doctorate (1824), in Vienna. Still under Emperor Franz I, Peithner was granted ad personam the privilege to treat his patients homeopathically.[113] Another pioneer of homeopathy in Bohemia was Dr Rudolph Schaller (1779 – 1857) who, until 1835, constantly lived in danger of being persecuted for violating the law that forbade homeopathy. He managed, however, to win a number of court cases because of his connections with influential circles in Prague.[114] A similarly important role was played in the 1830s by Dr Joseph Beer Ritter von Baier (1788 – 1857). He worked as a medical doctor in the Prague orphanage and later as personal physician to Prince Öttingen-Wallerstein. He also belonged to a small circle of individuals who broke the ground for homeopathy in Bohemia.[115] In the rural parts of mid-Bohemia, the homeopathic doctor Georg Rozischeck (1775 – 1856) of Votice (Wotitz) practised already in the 1820s. In 1830, he entered the service of Baron Riese-Stallburg as his personal homeopathic physician. Among the pioneers of homeopathy in Moravia was Dr Franz Hauptmann in Zasmuck (Zásmucky). He consulted Hahnemann in 1829 on how to treat a particular patient.[116] Of even greater importance was the aforementioned surgeon Anton Fischer who, already in 1818, tried to cure chronically ill patients with homeopathic remedies. He practised first in Rosice (Rossitz) and from 1825 onwards in Brno (Brünn). His influential clients included the Governor of Moravia and Silesia, Karl Rudolf Count Inzaghi (1777 – 1856) and General Ignaz Ludwig Paul Freiherr von Lederer (1769 – 1849). Rumour has it that even a judge who sentenced him for violating the law prohibiting homeopathy (which remained in force until 1835) consulted him as a doctor.[117] Persecution by the medical authorities forced Fischer to flee to the Benedictine monastery in Raigern (Rajhrad).[118] Another protagonist of homeopathy in Moravia was the lay healer Carl Steigentesch, a wealthy merchant in Brno. He had some training as a surgeon and owned a comprehensive homeopathic library.[119] He made good use of his excellent connections with influential society members in order to win more supporters for Hahnemann's doctrine. Together with another homeopathic practitioner in Brno, Dr Hože, Steigentesch travelled to Paris in 1840 in order to visit Hahnemann and to take part in the annual festivities of 10th August (the date of Hahnemann's doctorate). In Schönberg, a Moravian town famous for its textile manufacturing, the homeopathic surgeon Dominic Lauer had practised since 1825.[120] The first homeopathic physician to set up practice in Moravia was Adolph Heinrich Gerstel (1805 – 1890), a pupil of Hahnemann, who had treated cholera patients in Brno since 1831 and who continued to work as a medical practitioner and homeopath. In 1842, he relocated to Vienna where he joined the medical faculty.[121]

The great enthusiasm with which homeopathy was received in Brno at the beginning of the 1830s is shown by a letter that Hahnemann wrote in 1832 in which he says: 'The population of Brno is very much in favour of homeopathy.'[122] In northern Moravia it was predominantly the clergy who actively promoted homeopathy, with some clergymen even working as lay practitioners.[123]

The successful treatment of cholera in particular facilitated the breakthrough of homeopathy at the beginning of the 1830s, not only in Bohemia and Moravia. The English homeopath Frederick Forster Hervey Quin (1799 – 1879) arrived in 1831 in the small Moravian town of Tišnov in order to assist his colleagues Gerstel and Hanusch, who had become sick, with treating the numerous cholera patients in the town. According to the mayor of this town, Ernst Dieble, 680 of the 6671 inhabitants had contracted cholera. 331 of these patients were treated allopathically, but only 229 of these were cured. Of the 278 patients who received homeopathic therapy, apparently only 27 died.[124]

A directory[125] from the year 1860 registers one or even several homeopaths for each of the following Bohemian and Moravian towns: Budišovkou (Bautsch), Boskovice (Boskowitz), Polevsko (Blottendorf), Brno (Brünn), Most (Brüx), České Budějovice (Budweis), Chlumec nad Cidlinou (Chlumetz), Dobriz (near Prague), Velké Meziřiči (Grossmeseritsch), Lázně Jeleč (Geltschberg), Heřmanův Městec (Hermannstädtel), Dvorce (Hof), Jorice (Horschitz), Janowice (Janowitz), Jaromer (Jaromirsch), (Karlovy Vary (Karlsbad), Komotov (Kommotau), Česká Lípa (Leipa), Nechranice (Nechanitz), Olomouc (Olmütz), Postoloprty (Postelberg), Prostějov (Prossnitz), Lodenice (Pohrlitz), Hradčovice? (Radschütz=Radschowitz?), Rychnov na Moravě (Reichenau), Krásná Hora (Schönberg), Zduchovice (Sduchowitz), Štekeň nad Strakonice? (Stecken), Telc/Jihlava (Teltsch), Teplice (Teplitz), Terezín (Theresienstadt), Tišnov (Tischnowitz), Vejprty (Weipert), Odolena Voda (Wodolka), Zlonice (Zlonitz) and Znojmo (Znaim). Fourteen (!) homeopaths were practising in Prague alone at the time: Dr Salomon Duseny, Dr Altschul, Dr Hirsch, Dr Nathan Elsaß, Docent Dr Hofrichter, Dr Kafka, Dr Komareck, Dr Kovacz, Dr Michl, Dr Porges, Dr Seegen sen., Dr Seegen jun., Dr Teller, Dr Wehle. Towards the end of the 19th century there were considerably less. Already in 1864 people complained that the homeopathic practitioners were getting old and that new blood was needed in this profession.[126] An 1894 address register still mentions fourteen towns in Bohemia and Moravia where homeopathic doctors and surgeons were still active.[127] For Prague, however, there is only one entry: Dr Theodor Kafka. After World War I the number went down even further. In 1936, the Czech delegate to the LHMI estimated that there were only five homeopaths in his whole country. Homeopathy received another blow after 1945 when it was in the CSSR also banned as 'unscientific' and forced into an underground existence.

Together with Munich, Vienna and Leipzig, Prague was one of the first universities where homeopathy was officially allowed to be taught.[128] From 1850, Dr Elias Altschul lectured in the medical faculty of this university on homeopathy.[129] This lectureship came with a polyclinic which essentially consisted in Dr Altschul's private practice. In 1860, he organised a public final examination for the graduates of his course, in which Professor Joseph Halla (1814 – 1887) participated who was then Dean of the Medical Faculty at the Charles University.[130] Although his lectures were, on the whole, not that well frequented, Dr Altschul was greatly respected by his faculty colleagues because of his outstanding expertise. His funeral was attended not only by the president but also by the dean of the medical faculty.[131] Franz Josef Hofrichter (1803 – 1883) also lectured here on special therapy and homeopathy from 1851 onwards until his death.[132]

Since the 1880s homeopathy has not been represented again at any of the Czech universities.[133] German pharmaceutical companies started to offer introductory courses for homeopathy in the 1930s.[134] This tradition was followed up in the early 1990s when an Austrian pharmaceutical company supported training courses for homeopathic physicians in Kroměříž (Kremsier).[135] Today, homeopaths are trained in three-year-courses which the Czech Medical Homeopathic Association has offered since 1999. Admission to the School of Classical Homeopathy which was founded by the publisher Alternativa in Prague and cooperates with the Faculty of Homeopathy in London is not restricted anymore to medical doctors. There are also training courses in Brno.[136]

The Czech Republic looks back on a long tradition of homeopathic hospitals which was, however, interrupted towards the end of the 19th century and has, up to the present time, not been revived again. Around 1850, there was, for example, a hospital for the poor in Nechranice (Nechanitz) which was founded in 1846 by Marie Therese Countess of Harrach (1771 – 1852). Its director was a certain Dr Feltl and between 1846 and 1848 a total of 404 patients were treated homeopathically there. The mortality rate was around 2.5 percent.[137] This institution is also mentioned in the address register of 1860.[138] Apart from that, there existed in the 1850s Dr Altschul's polyclinic (without beds) in Prague which has been mentioned already as well as a homeopathic hospital run by the Sisters of Mercy in Kroměřiž (Kremsier). Head of this hospital in the 1840s was a certain Dr Schweitzer. In the revolution year 1848 altogether 472 inpatients and 516 outpatients were treated here homeopathically.[139] At the beginning of the 1860s homeopathic treatment was introduced in the municipal hospital in Most (Brüx) following a resolution of the district council. A homeopathic physician (Dr Karl Müller) had been practising there already since 1840. In the Moravian town of Zwitta a homeopathic hospital opened in 1868, but nothing more is known about its history.[140] The same applies to the small homeopathic 12-bed-hospital in Zleb, whose benefactress was Princess Wilhelmine Auersperg who put her physician, Dr Kohout, in charge.[141]

As early as 1835, that is earlier than in all the other Austrian territories, homeopaths were granted permission to practise and, more importantly, to dispense in Bohemia and Moravia.[142] This was preceded by an inquiry directed to the Medical School at the University in Prague on 6th June 1834, with the question if homeopathy could be considered to be a scientific system.[143] As the experts returned a positive answer homeopaths were now free to practise and on 10th February 1837 the law that had previously prohibited homeopathy was finally abolished in all 'hereditary lands'.[144] In 1846, a new decision of the court chancery granted homeopaths a restricted right of dispensary which, in 1857, was further specified with a decree from the Ministry of Justice in Vienna.[145] An edict of 1887 restricted the right to dispense to physicians who treated their patients exclusively with homeopathy and who adhered strictly to the principles of potentisation. In Bohemia an edict from the governor in 1894 stipulated strict adherence to the relevant regulations and referred to cases of abuse. One year later, another edict, issued by the same authority, ruled that all physicians who had permission to keep their own dispensary should procure their medical preparations, if possible, from the nearest pharmacy and keep an account on which homeopathic remedies were administered to which patients in which form.[146]

In the 1840s Prague was considered the key location in Europe for the manufacture of homeopathic first-aid kits. The precision with which the small glass vials were produced was particularly praised at the time.[147] The first public homeopathic pharmacy opened in 1860 in Prague[148] and in 1894 there were already two: 'Engel' and 'Zum weißen Einhorn'(The white unicorn). At the beginning of the 1890s homeopathic pharmacies appeared also in other Bohemian and Moravian towns, for example in Komotov[149] as the right of dispensary was not restricted any longer. In the 1930s the companies Dr Schwabe and Madaus opened branches in Teplice and Liberec. In 1931, Schwabe exported homeopathic remedies worth 19,600 Reichsmark into what was then Czechoslovakia. After the occupation of the Sudetenland the Liberec[150] branch was liquidated. After that, homeopaths bought their homeopathic remedies wholesale.[151] Even today, with homeopathy experiencing a renaissance in the Czech Republic, foreign companies are supplying the homeopathic medicines.

In the 1930s no homeopathic veterinary doctors were known in Czechoslovakia[152], and this in spite of the fact that animal homeopathy in Bohemia and Moravia goes back as far as the 1830s. A pioneer on this field was Dr R. Löw, who worked in Dražovice (Domoraz) and the surrounding villages. He published his cases later on in the *Prager Monatsschrift für Homöopathie* (Prague Monthly Journal for Homeopathy).[153] The homeopathic surgeon Dr Florian Sirsch in Šumperk (Schönberg) occasionally also treated animals.[154]

As with the German states, homeopathy in the Czech Republic owes its breakthrough in the first half of the 19th century to the success of the cholera therapy in the 1830s and 1840s. Apart from that, homeopathy had influential supporters, especially members of the aristocracy, who consulted homeopathic physicians.[155] The Princes Windischgrätz and Lamberg zu Zusiowitz both kept homeopaths as their personal physicians. In the second half, however, homeopathy became less important, especially in the towns where the scientific medical approach had grown into a strong opposition. After World War II the CSSR remained for a long time under Soviet influence which means that homeopathy was struggling due to constant prohibitions and bureaucratic chicanery. After the fall of the Iron Curtain homeopathy experienced a new boost in the area of the former Czechoslovakia which is still noticeable today. Among the persons who fought for the homeopathic cause in the early 1990s was the homeopathic physician Princess of Schwarzenberg whose famous ancestor, the war hero of the Battle of Leipzig in 1813, was one of Hahnemann's prominent patients.

Slovakia

During negotiations between the Slovak leaders and the Czech part of the republic the decision was taken in 1993 to divide the Czechoslovak Federation into two independent states. Since 1st May 2004 Slovakia – just as the Czech Republic – has been an EU member. Even though the former two parts of one country are now going their own national ways, they still look back over a common history that stretches over many centuries: first within the Habsburg monarchy and then as the Republic of Czechoslovakia. The history of homeopathy is also in many ways similar and still today Slovak homeopaths are reading their medical literature in the Czech language.

That all the classics of homeopathy, starting from Hahnemann's writings and the repertories of Boenninghausen and Rückert to Hering's drug provings were widely read in their original language in what is now Slovakia (this includes the territories that used to belong to Upper Hungary), is documented in the letters that the Austrian homeopath Joseph Attomyr (1807 – 1856) wrote while staying in Bratislava and published in Leipzig in 1833/34.[156] He also subscribed to German homeopathic journals. It can be assumed that he was not the only German speaking homeopath to have access to the relevant literature in this part of the Habsburg monarchy and to keep informed by reading journals and corresponding with colleagues. Translations of fundamental homeopathic works into Czech or Slovakian only became necessary when the traditional bond with the German speaking countries weakened and the national movement started to employ active language policies. There are, however, still no Slovak homeopathic journals today, but, at least, some of the works of Jan Scholten and Rajan Sankaran are now available in the Slovak language.[157]

During the 19th century the homeopathic doctors who were practising in what is now Slovakia, were mostly members of the Austrian Homeopathic Physicians' Association which was founded in 1846. The membership list of 1862 names two homeopaths in Bratislava: Dr Anton Eduard Nehrer and Dr Ábrahám von Szontagh (1830 – 1902).[158] The latter was, as an 1857 news release informs us, personal physician of Count J.N. Zichy in Bratislava. Later on he settled in Pest and became secretary of the Hungarian Homeopathic Doctors' Association.[159] The Slovak Homeopathic Society was only founded in 1991 and counts not only doctors but also pharmacists amongst its members. In the year 2001 this association had 360 members. In 1997, another association of Slovak homeopaths (Slovak Homeopathic Chamber) was initiated by the French manufacturer of homeopathic remedies, Boiron. By 1998, its membership had already risen to sixty.[160] For a few years now there has also existed a homeopathic lay organisation.[161]

One of the pioneers of homeopathy in Slovakia was without doubt the aforementioned Dr Attomyr.[162] He had gained his doctorate in Munich in 1831 with a medical dissertation on *Quaedam quodad psychiatriam homeopathicam* and had contact with Hahnemann. Homeopathy had been introduced to him already in 1825 by the Austrian regimental doctor Dr J. Müller. In 1832, Attomyr became personal physician to Count Csáky, whom he accompanied on several of his journeys. For a relatively short period of time he worked as a physician in Levoča (Leutschau), which, in 1840, became the centre of the Slovak national movement. In 1833, he travelled with the count to the opening of parliament in Bratislava, where he remained until his appointment as family physician to the Duke of Lucca. In his *Letters on Homeopathy* he describes his homeopathic practice and alludes to an extensive personal homeopathic pharmacy, which included 125 to 150 of the most commonly used remedies. He even offered to sell these remedies (in D30 or higher potency) at low cost to interested laypersons and doctors, in order to propagate homeopathy.[163] In 1833, he managed to convince over 20 wealthy 'friends of homeopathy in this area'[164] to donate money to the newly founded Homeopathic Hospital in Leipzig. After his return from Lucca and a short stay in Spiš (Zips) Attomyr lived in Bratislava again, from where he moved to the Hungarian town of Pest. In 1844/45 he finally settled in Bratislava and practised there until his death. According to the report of a travelling French homeopath[165], a few years before Attomyr's arrival, another homeopath named Loebell was active in Bratislava and also a homeopathic surgeon called Anneli [recte: Haneli].

Around 1860, Bratislava was already a stronghold of homeopathy. A directory from that year lists eight homeopathic doctors and surgeons in this town alone: Dr Franz Cservinka, Dr Ritter von Koch, Dr Nehrer, surgeon Setéth, Dr Sigmann, Dr Streibig, Dr v. Szontagh, surgeon Weißweiler. Only two are documented, however, in 1894 in Bratislava; and just before World War I only one was left.[166] Apart from that homeopathic doctors are mentioned in a few other towns that now belong to Slovakia. In Košice a certain Dr Kain practised in 1860, and, at the beginning of the 1890s, Dr Felix Parcher, who still worked there shortly before World War I.

In contrast to the Czech Republic, Slovakia never had a lectureship for homeopathy. With the dissolution of the Czechoslovak federation at the beginning of the 1990s, non-university training courses for homeopathy were set up in Slovakia. As in the Czech Republic these were run by the different homeopathic associations. From 1992 to 1996, there was even a Centre for Homeopathy at the Institute for Post-Graduate Education for Doctors and Pharmacists in Bratislava which, however, was closed down again due to pressure from the Slovak Doctors' Association. Until now, homeopathy has also not succeeded in entering the three medical schools in the country because there is too much resistance.[167]

Just as in other territories that were under Habsburg rule in the 19th century, homeopathic doctors in the areas which now belong to Slovakia and used to be part of Upper Hungary, were granted legal permission to practise freely and shortly afterwards also the right of restricted dispensary. Around the year 1894 there was a homeopathic pharmacy in Košice ('Zum Auge Gottes' – Eye of God).[168] It is not known if there were other institutions like that in the country. Since 1998 homeopathic remedies are officially permitted in Slovakia on the basis of the 'Act about Medicines and Medical Products, No 40/1998'. In 1999, homeopathic remedies were available in about a third of over 300 pharmacies in the country.[169] To this day there is no pharmaceutical company in Slovakia that manufactures homeopathic medicines so they have to be imported from abroad.

That veterinary homeopathy has been practised for a long time in Slovakia is shown by the fact that Attomyr used homeopathic methods against the cattle plague (Löserdürre) on Count Csáky's farms in 1837.[170]

As in the Czech Republic homeopathy was mostly taboo in Slovakia until the end of the communist era. There were no training possibilities for newcomers and it was difficult to obtain homeopathic remedies. Even today it only plays a part in private practice.

Hungary

All the pioneers of homeopathy in Hungary were German-speaking and some of them owned comprehensive libraries. As early as 1830 the fourth edition of Hahnemann's *Organon* came out in Hungarian in a translation by Pál Bugát and József Horváth.[171] In 1863, János Garay published his medical dissertation in Hungarian under the title *Értekezés a homeopathikus gyógy-és gyógyszertanról és adagokról* (A Contribution to Homeopathy, Remedies and Dosage). The book gives an outline of the homeopathic theory and supplies contemporary scientific evidence of the effectiveness of homeopathic remedies. It also contains a medicinal study of the blue monkshood *(Értekezés a sisakvirágról/Aconit)*. During the first half of the 20th century only few fundamental works on homeopathy came out in Hungarian as the number of interested homeopaths had gone down dramatically. One exception is Gustav Schimert's book *Allopathia és Homeopathia* (Allopathy and Homeopathy, Budapest 1928).[172] Since the end of the 1990s many important foreign repertories and pharmacologies have been available in Hungarian translation, among others *Farmakológia és homeopátiás matéria medica* by Denis Demarque et al. (Budapest, 1999).

Introductions to homeopathy that were aimed at laypersons spread particularly fast. In 1847, the homeopathic physician Döme (Demetrius) Argenti (1809 – 1893) published a book with the title *Homöopathische Behandlung verschiedener Krankheiten* (Homeopathic treatment of various illnesses) of which eight Hungarian and two German editions came out and over 10,000 copies were sold.[173] Other popular guidebooks for laymen followed soon in Hungarian: András Ivanovich, *A hasonszenvi házi és úti orvos, vagyis a tanácsadó kisebb és sürgetöbb bajokban* (Homeopathic family practitioner for home and abroad and guidelines for minor and major illnesses), 1837; Imre Lovász, *Mit tartsunk a Homeoopathiáról* (What do people think of homeopathy?), 1838. In the second half of the 19th century another book by Döme Argenti came out under the title *Hasonszenvi utitárs rögtön támadt betegségek elhárítására* (Homeopathic companion for the treatment of acute acquired illnesses), Pest 1863. Because his writings were so popular, not many new books were published for laypersons in the second half of the 19th century. In 1862, a book by Clothar Müller came out in Hungarian which became very successful. It was called *Hasonszenvi házi s családi orvos* (The homeopathic family doctor). An introduction to homeopathy by Tilhamér Balogh von Almás (1838 – 1907) appeared in 1889 with a second edition following in 1904 under the title *Elsö segedelem hirtelen elöforduló betegségekés baleseteknél a homöopathák eljárása szerint* (First Aid in cases of acutely acquired illnesses and accidents according to the homeopathic practice).

The extent to which these publications contributed to the popularisation of homeopathy in Hungary should not be underestimated. They were easily accessible guidebooks which were particularly popular among clergymen and teachers who, next to members of the aristocracy, were most instrumental in promoting the homeopathic movement, especially in rural areas.

The first homeopathic journal in Hungarian appeared on 1st July 1864. The editor of this monthly paper (*Hasonszenvi Közlöny* – Homeopathic Newsletter) was Stefan Horner (Vezekényi), who was also in charge of the homeopathic hospital in Gyöngyös. It was, however, discontinued after only one year[174] and replaced in 1866 by *Hasonszenvi lapok* (Notes on Homeopathy) which were copy-edited by Ábrahám von Szontagh and came out in Pest until 1876. From 1895 to 1900 the journal *Homeopathia* was published with Bakody as chief editor.[175] A congress periodical which was published for the first time in 1935 ceased to appear already one year later. Since the 1990s Hungary has had its own homeopathic journal again: SIMILE.

In 1843 Hungarian homeopaths made their first attempt at forming an association.[176] Initiators were Josef Attomyr, who by then already practised in Pest, and Carl Heinrich Rosenberg, who was personal physician to Count Batthyány. The small but nevertheless very presentable number of homeopaths in the country had, however, reservations with regard to this scheme, and the political climate, i.e. the looming Hungarian liberation fights of 1848/49, was not exactly conducive to this kind of endeavour. In 1863, another appeal was launched for the foundation of a homeopathic association that should, however, not admit laypersons. This time the initiators were, among others, Tivadar Bakody, János Garay, Ferenc (Franz) Hausmann (1811 – 1876) and Ábrahám von Szontagh. An association was founded on 28th December 1865.[177] By the end of 1874 the membership of the Hungarian homeopathic doctors' association (Magyar Hasonszenvi Orvosegylet) had risen to 40, of which 21 resided in Budapest or close by. The first chairman was Pál Almási Balogh (1794 – 1867). With the death of the last chairman, Tivadar Bakody, in 1911 the work of the association came to a standstill, although it officially only ceased to exist in 1949. Only in 1991 a new homeopathic society was founded which also became a LHMI member.[178] This union counted nearly 300 members in 2001, among them 177 physicians and 28 veterinary doctors, as well as 28 dentists and 66 pharmacists.[179]

According to Rosenberg there were already 85 homeopathic physicians in Hungary in 1843, with as many as ten of them practising in Pest.[180] For the year 1860 an address list registers, by name, 38 homeopathic physicians and surgeons for the Kingdom of Hungary.[181] At the beginning of the 1870s Balogh estimated that there were around 40 to 50 homeopathic doctors in the country. He thought, however, that the rural areas were undersupplied.[182] According to a later address directory only fourteen were left in 1894.[183] Shortly before World War I, 20 homeopaths were listed in an international address directory.[184] In 1931, there were only 10 practitioners in the whole country.[185] A few years later, in 1935, the number had already risen to 50 again[186] and nowadays there are several hundred homeopaths in Hungary.

Hungary belongs to those countries where homeopathic hospitals were set up very early.[187] The first of them opened in a provincial town. Already at the beginning of the 1820s patients were treated homeopathically in the 'Care Home for the Mentally Ill' in Nagyvárad (Großwardein), which today belongs to Romania.[188] Using his own means and donations a doctor started a homeopathic hospital in Kőszeg (Güns) in 1833. It had 24 beds and one room for the treatment of outpatients. 738 patients were treated homeopathically here between 1833 and 1841 and the mortality rate is said to have been as low as 4%.[189] Another homeopathic hospital opened in Gyöngyös in 1838 with the financial support of Baroness Orczy.[190] It had also a surgical department and started with 24 beds, but the number of patients increased over the years. In 1857 this private hospital passed into public ownership. Following a short interplay with a new director who preferred the allopathic approach, homeopathy won the day and 120 patients were treated here in 1872. Senior physician was for many decades Dr Stephan Horner (Vezekényi, 1808 – 1891) whom we met already in his position as editor. In 1844, homeopathy was introduced into the prison hospital in Miskolc. Because it proved very successful its application was extended to include the poor in the area. After only one year and a quarter, however, this experiment was discontinued due to pressure from the medical establishment. The head of the institution, Dr Lipót Stern, continued to practise as a homeopathic doctor in Miskolc. In 1866, the first homeopathic hospital opened in Pest. Initiator and later also director of this privately funded institution was Dr Tivadar Bakody (1825 – 1911). In 1872, the Bethesda Hospital moved into the Bartl Palace on Hermina Straße. 11,305 patients received homeopathic therapy here between 1882 and 1897. In 1870 the second hospital for homeopathy opened its gates in Pest. Its benefactress was Countess Zichy (née von Metternich!). The hospital which was named after Elisabeth Queen of Hungary had 12 beds and was first situated on Fö-Straße (later Fö-Knézich-Straße) in the Pest district of Franzstadt. Its first medical director was Dr Ferenc (Franz) Hausmann and the nurses were nuns from the order of the Sisters of Mercy.[191] 7,952 patients received homeopathic treatment here between 1884 and 1898.[192] In Theresienstadt, another quarter of Pest, the Hungarian Homeopathic Doctors' Association had operated a polyclinic since 1867 where surgery was held three times a week.[193] In its first year 314 patients were treated here.[194] In Esztergom (Gran) there was also a homeopathic hospital in the 1870s which had 30 beds. Its director was Dr Lörinczy.[195] Dr Bakody who has been mentioned already became director of a homeopathic ward in the St. Rochus Hospital in Pest, where the Emperor paid an official visit in 1876 and used the opportunity to inform himself about homeopathic treatment.[196] This clinic treated as many as 46,485 patients between 1871 and 1897.[197] In the 1930s only one homeopathic hospital was left in the entire country: the Elisabeth-Spital. It had 10 beds and its director was Dr Gustav Schimert.[198]

Already in 1844 homeopaths called for the establishment of an academic chair for the new medical approach at the University in Pest but the emperor turned down their application.[199] When the physician Dr János Garay applied to the medical faculty of the University in Pest to be appointed 'private lecturer on homeopathy' his request was still flatly refused. He received, however, permission to publish his dissertation on homeopathic pharmacology. One of the aims of the Hungarian Homeopathic Doctors' Association was to introduce homeopathy into the medical schools. Already in 1867, at the time of the Austrian-Hungarian Settlement, petitions were addressed to the Home and Education Secretary demanding equality with allopathy in research and tuition.[200] The homeopaths benefited from the fact that many important leaders of the Hungarian Liberation Fight, for example István Széchenyi, belonged to their clientele. It took nevertheless three years until their efforts were crowned with success. With a majority decision in 1870 the Hungarian parliament endorsed the establishment of an academic chair at the University of Pest and of a public homeopathic hospital.[201] In 1871 the first chair, which was more therapy-based, was occupied by Ferenc (Franz) Hausmann who had had many years' experience as medical director of a homeopathic hospital. After his death

(1876) the chair was not re-occupied. A second professorship with emphasis on theory was added in 1873. It was occupied by Theodor von Bakody (1825 – 1911). Bakody did not have a successor either, but he remained lecturer at the university for over 31 years. He never had many students, though, as most of them did not dare to defy the threats of the medical school's allopathic fraction. In this respect, the apprehensions of the former editor of the *Allgemeine Homöopathische Zeitung* (General Homeopathic Journal), Arnold Lorbacher (1818 – 1899), proved true: that the appointment of a homeopath as university professor was comparable to the appointment of a protestant theologian in a predominantly catholic faculty. The rise in prestige was therefore ultimately not sufficient to secure the urgently needed younger generation of homeopaths. This meant that towards the end of the 19th century homeopathy in Hungary experienced a deep crisis from which it did not recover for many decades.

Despite the fact that homeopathy was so popular in this country, the leading homeopaths of the *Gründerzeit* [202] were acutely aware that, due to the lack of new practitioners, its future was severely jeopardised. By the mid-1930s homeopathy had been pushed out of the universities.[203] There were only training courses run by Dr Margittai and Dr Macskássy.[204] Since the renaissance of homeopathy in Hungary in the 1990s efforts have been made to bring homeopathy back into the medical schools, but this endeavour has not been altogether successful. A draft law from 1870 concerning the tuition of homeopathy at Pest University already had similar objectives.[205] What has been achieved up to now is that certified homeopathy courses are offered at the faculties of veterinary medicine.[206]

In 1876, the Hungarian homeopaths were granted the right of dispensary, but they had to commit themselves to procure the original substances from a pharmacy and to give the potentiated medicines to patients free of charge.[207] There is evidence that homeopathic drugs were sold in a pharmacy in Pest as early as 1837.[208] Some Hungarian homeopaths got their medical supply from a priest name Trunessek who was also a popular healer.[209] Since 1858 there had been one homeopathic pharmacy in the country, that of pharmacist Jarmay in Pest.[210] At the beginning of the 1930s the number had risen to three: the pharmacies Engel, Szentcsalád and Zoltán. The latter was a branch of the company Willmar Schwabe in Leipzig.[211] In 1934, the German company Madaus (based in Radebeul) opened a branch in Budapest which supplied a web of affiliated pharmacies in Hungary. Since the 1990s Dr Peithner Ltd. (Vienna) along with Biologische Heilmittel Heel GmbH (Baden-Baden) have been important suppliers of homeopathic and phytotherapeutic products to the Hungarian market.

In 1837, the prohibition of homeopathic practice was abolished in the Kingdom of Hungary.[212] A number of physicians had, however, managed before already to bypass this law, because they were, like Dr Josef von Bakody (1795 – 1845), family physicians of influential families. Because of the successful treatment of cholera, for which there was plenty of evidence, homeopathy had won over the population, including many politicians and civil servants.[213] After a long time of flourishing the decline came at the beginning of the 20th century, interrupted by a short phase of revival in the mid-1930s. From 1948 to the fall of the Iron Curtain homeopathy in Hungary, as in other Eastern European states, was prohibited and frowned upon. Since

1997[214] homeopathy has been officially recognized again. It is not integrated in the national health system but some private health insurers are now paying for treatment. This development was preceded by the employment of homeopathic doctors by sickness funds in the 1870s.[215]

In 1857, Friedrich August Günther's book on veterinary homeopathy *(Hasonszenvi állatorvos)* came out in Arad, translated by the solicitor Imre Náray. It is said to have sold 200 copies within eight days of its publication.[216] Károly Böhm's book *Közhasznú hasonszenvi állatorvosi könyv* (Handbook for homeopathic veterinary medicine) came out in 1864, and one year later György Hübner's *Hasonszenvi házi állatorvos* (Veterinary homeopathy at home). The homeopathic newsletter *Hasonszenvi lapok* that was published from 1866 to 1876 included a regular page on veterinary homeopathy from 1871 onwards.[217] The specialised diploma-courses that are offered nowadays by the veterinary faculties of Hungarian universities are continuing this tradition of homeopathic health care for animals.

Greece

Greece became part of the Ottoman Empire in 1453. In 1821, its fight for liberation began and led ultimately to an independence that was guaranteed in the London Protocol of 3rd February 1830. This state comprised, however, only the smaller part of modern-day Greece. Thessalia, for example, was only acquired in 1881, Crete in 1908. Most islands as well as Epirus in the Northwest and large parts of Macedonia (with Thessaloniki) became only Greek after the Balkan Wars of 1912/13.

Hahnemann's *Organon* was not translated into the Greek language until 1989. Before that, in 1969, George Vithoulkas' introduction to homeopathy *(Homeopathy - Medicine of the New Man)* was published in Athens and shortly afterwards translated into many languages. It became a bestseller. Today many other fundamental writings on homeopathy are available in the Greek language. Since the mid-1970s there has also been a Greek homeopathic journal (*Omoiopathitiki Iatrik*, 1974 ff.)[218] which is published in Athens.

Homeopathy did not succeed in gaining ground in Greece during the 19th century, neither under the Ottoman Empire nor after the declaration of independence in 1830. In the 1840s there seems to have been a homeopathic doctor in Athens called Tabini, who had previously been unknown. He is said to have moved in higher society circles and to have benefited from the active support of the Austrian Ambassador in Greece, Anton Count Prokesch-Osten (1795 – 1876).[219] The discussion in other countries about the new medical approach certainly also found interest in the Greek Kingdom. Towards the end of the 1850s a Greek medical journal alludes to a court case in Paris that had to do with homeopathy.[220] Already in 1831 a foreign journal reported that sick people had been treated homeopathically during the cholera epidemic in Constantinople by two German doctors who lived in the city on the Bosporus.[221] At the beginning of the 1840s five homeopathic doctors are said to have practised in Istanbul (Untersberg, Tomaszwesky, Lutzy, Berson and Macabini).[222] Smyrna (now Izmir) which was ceded to Greece in the 1920 Treaty of Sèvres, but freed again two years later, did not possess a single homeopathic doctor in the mid-19th century. Only in Istanbul a French doctor tried his hand, among other things, at homeopathy without knowing too much about it, as reported by an English Consul in the year 1851. 'In the annals of homeopathy Turkey must still be blank', reads a letter to the editor of the *British Journal of Homeopathy*. The writer also points out that there were two other Greek doctors inland who had some interest in homeopathy and to whom he had sent relevant reading material. Any efforts to convince European doctors to come and settle in the Greek speaking part of Asia Minor had apparently failed. The report ends with the words: 'Had I time I should translate into Greek some elementary works.' [223] Before World War I an American homeopath worked in Istanbul who held his surgery in English.[224]

Before 1965, there were only a few homeopathic doctors in Greece; among them was Ioannis Pikramenos (1880 – 1971) who had a practice in Athens and whom his patients held in high esteem because of his healing successes. He was a graduate doctor but self taught in homeopathy. He acquired his knowledge prevalently from the journal *L'Homéopathie française* which had been founded in 1912 by the French homeopath Dr Léon Vannier (1880 – 1963).

After graduating from the medical school of Athens University in 1906 Pikramenos spent five years in France and then moved to Egypt where he worked as a medical doctor. In 1931, he returned to Greece where he opened a homeopathic practice in 1933 which he kept till the end of the 1960s. He procured homeopathic medicines from France, but also produced them himself.[225] Only in 1959 the pharmacist Pavlos Tsivanidis began to produce and import homeopathic remedies.

The history of homeopathy in Greece really only started in the 1960s when homeopath George Vithoulkas who had been trained in India and South Africa returned to his country and offered training courses for interested doctors. These courses soon became very popular. In 1969, homeopathy was so established in Greece, that it was decided to hold the Liga-Congress in Athens. In 1970, the Athenian School of Homeopathic Medicine was founded and one year later another one followed: The Hellenic Homeopathic Medical Society (H.H.M.S.). This society organises further training seminars and has held an annual congress since 1983.[226] Since 1975 it has been a member of LHMI and in 1998 it counted 125 members.[227]

According to the *World Dictionary* the number of homeopaths in Greece was 18 at the beginning of the 1970s.[228] In 1995, it had apparently already risen to 130.[229]

Since 1995 training for homeopaths has not just been available in the school in Athens but also at the International Academy for Classical Homeopathy. George Vithoulkas who received the Alternative Nobel Price in 1996, had founded the Academy on the island of Alonissos. In 1993, the Hippocratean Center of Classical

Homeopathy opened in Athens and welcomes students who have not graduated in medicine. Its president is Gerasimos Stouraitis who also founded the Homeopathic Association of Hellas in 1997 which is a member of ECCH.[230]

At the end of the 1990s there were already five homeopathic polyclinics.[231] The relevant literature does not supply any information about the number of homeopathic pharmacies. How much the interest in homeopathy has risen over the last years is shown by the fact that, initiated by a former Greek ambassador, an exhibition about the history of homeopathy was hosted by the Goethe Institute in Athens.[232]

Notes

[1] Martin Dinges (ed.), *Weltgeschichte der Homöopathie. Länder, Schulen, Heilkundige* (Munich, 1996), p. 15.

[2] Alexander Kotok, *The history of homeopathy in the Russian Empire until World War I, as compared with other European countries and the USA: similarities and discrepancies* (Ph. D. dissertation, Hebrew University Jerusalem, 1999), http://homeoint.org/books4/kotok/; Alexander Kotok, Medical heresy struggles for the right on 'otherness': homeopathy in the USSR, forthcoming in *Medizin, Gesellschaft und Geschichte (MedGG)* 25 (2007).

[3] Nena Zidov, An Overview of the History of Homeopathy in Slovenia in the 19th century. In: *MedGG* 23 (2005), pp. 181-198.

[4] Alexander Kotok, Homeopathy in Bulgaria: from revolutionaries to professionals. In: *Orvostörténeti Közlemények (Communicationes de historia artis medicinae)* 186/87 (2004), pp. 131-137.

[5] Erika Koltay, History of alternative medicine in Hungary in 19th and early 20th century. In: *Orvostörténeti Közlemények (Communicationes de historia artis medicinae)* 188/89 (2004), pp. 57-68; Maria Kócián/ Lívia Kölnei, The Struggle of Gustav Schimert for the Revival of Homeopathy in Hungary (1908-1944). In: *Orvostörténeti Közlemények (Communicationes de historia artis medicinae)* 188/89 (2004), pp. 101-106; Mária Kócián Lívia Kölnei, Geschichte der Homöopathie in Ungarn (1820-1871). In: *MedGG 23* (2005), pp. 201-212.

[6] Sigriur Svana Pétursdóttir, Homoeopathy in Iceland. In: *Historical Aspects of Unconventional Medicine. Approaches, Concepts, Case Studies*, edited by Robert Jütte, Motzi Eklöf, Marie Nelson (Sheffield, 2001), pp. 183-192.

[7] Fernando Dario Francois Flores, History of the Homeopathic Medicine in Mexico, 1849-2001. In: *MedGG* 23 (2005), pp. 217-240; Heinz Eppenich, Malaische Identität und Islamisierung der Homöopathie in Malaysia. In: *MedGG* 17 (1999), pp. 149-176.

[8] Julian Winston, *The Faces of Homeopathy. An illustrated history of the first 200 years*. (Tawa/New Zealand, 1999); Eswara Das, *History & Status of Homeopathy around the World* (New Delhi, 2005).

[9] http://www.homeopathyhome.com/reference/articles/ukhomhistory.shtml.

[10] Vgl. Oivind Larsen (ed.), *Norges Leger* (Oslo, 1996), vol. III, p. 301, vol. V, p. 57.

[11] V. Meyer (ed.); *Homöopathischer Führer für Deutschland und das gesamte Ausland* (Leipzig, 1860), p 126. Cf. Larsen (fn. 9), vol. V, p. 123.

[12] Fritz Donner, Über die gegenwärtige Lage der Homöopathie in Europa. In: *Allgemeine Homöopathische Zeitung (AHZ)* 179 (1931), pp. 229-271, especially p. 237.

[13] O. Farstad, L' homeopathie en Norvège. In: *Actes du Congrès*, LMHI (Geneva, 1931), pp. 57-58.

[14] Øyvind Schjelderup, *Homeopathic History of Norway* (http://www.geocities.com/klassiskhomeopati/history). See also Grethe Wien, Homeopatiens historie i Norge. In: *Dynamis*, issue no. 4 (1990), issue no. 1 (1991).

[15] Farstad (fn. 13), pp. 57-58.

[16] http://www.wholehealthnow.com/homeopathy_pro/norway.html.
[17] Schjelderup (fn. 14).
[18] E. J. Pedersen/ A. J. Norheim/ V. Fonnebe, Attitudes of Norwegian physicians to homeopathy. A questionnaire among 2,019 physicians on their cooperation with homeopathy specialists (in Norwegian). In: *Tidsskrift for Den Norsk Laegeforen* 116 (1996), pp. 2186-9.
[19] If not stated otherwise, the following information is according to H. W. Sjögren, Die Homöopathie in Schweden. In: *AHZ* 164 (1916), pp. 5-10; H. W. Sjögren, Die Homöopathie in Schweden 100 Jahre. In: *AHZ* 174 (1926), pp. 63-67, Winston (fn. 8), pp. 579-580.
[20] Per Jacob Liedbeck, *Homöopathiens närvarande ställning i främmande länder* (Stockholm, 1854; Per Jacob Liedbeck, *Homöopatiska polykliniken i Stockholm, oktober-december 1868* (Stockholm, 1869); Per Jacob Liedbeck, *Om kamfersprit allena, ett bepröfvadt koleramedel* (2nd ed., Stockholm, 1866).
[21] Fredrik Johansson, *Homeopatisk läkemedelshandbok (homeopatisk läkemedelslära) grundad på likhetslagen, similia similibus curantur* (Stockholm, 1923).
[22] Karl Stauffer, *Homeopatisk handbok* (Göteborg, 1983).
[23] James Tyler Kent, *Forelesninger i homøopatisk materia medica: 41 middel*, översatt och tillrättalagd på norska av Petter o. Ivan Lyngsgård (Göteborg, 1982); George Vithoulkas, Materia medica viva. Vol. 1: *Abelmoschus till Ambrosia artemisiae folia*, översättning Anita Back, Lars Sandwall Mölndal (Göteborg, 2002); Birgitta Sivermark-Wedberg, *Materia medica: homeopatisk läkemedelslära* (Helsingborg, 1997).
[24] *The International Homoeopathic Medical Directory 1911-12*, edited by J. Robertson Day, E. Petrie Hoyle (London, [1912]), p. 130.
[25] *Sitzungsberichte des X. Kongresses der Liga Homoepathica Internationalis in Budapest 19.-25. August 1935* (Radebeul/Dresden, [1935]), p. 463.
[26] Donner (ft. 12), p. 238.
[27] Vgl. http://www.lmhint.net/LigaLetter/March00/.
[28] http://www.kam.se/html/terapier/homeopatikagruppen/ in_english/030316_treatment_in_sweden_with_homeopathic_remedies.pdf. For the historical background, see Motzi Eklöf, Doctor or Quack. Legal and Lexical Definitions in Twentieth-Century Sweden. In: *Historical Aspects of Unconventional Medicine. Approaches, Concepts, Case Studies*, ed. by Robert Jütte, Motzi Eklöf, Marie Nelson (Sheffield, 2001), pp. 103-117.
[29] KAM = The Committee for Alternative Medicine, Sweden, cf. www.kam.se.
[30] See the resolution to the Swedish King, *11th Congress Liga Homoeopathica Internationalis.* (Glasgow, [1936]), p. 97.
[31] If not stated otherwise, the following information is according to Anna-Elisabeth Brade, Die Welt der Medizin und die Haltung der Legislative: Dänemark. In: Martin Dinges (ed.), *Weltgeschichte der Homöopathie* (Munich, 1996), pp. 132-154; and to Oskar Hansen, Geschichte der Homöopathie in Dänemark. In: *Berliner Homöopathische Zeitung* 4 (1885), pp. 327-335.
[32] Cf. Jacques Baur, *Ein Buch geht um die Welt. Die kleine Geschichte des Organon des Dr. Ch. F. Samuel Hahnemann*, übersetzt von Wolfgang Schweizer (Heidelberg, 1979), p. 29.

[33] Carl Otto, Oversigt af de i Aaret 1828 i Tugt= Rasp= og Forbedringshuset behandlede Syge; med Bemaerkninger om deres Behandlingsmaade. In: *Bibliotek for Laeger* (1829), pp. 246-252, especially p. 251.
[34] Cf. Michael Stolberg, Die Homöopathie auf dem Prüfstein. Der erste Doppelblindversuch der Medizingeschichte im Jahr 1835. In: *Münchener medizinische Wochenschrift* 138 (1996), pp. 364-366. On early clinical trials in homeopathy, see also Michael Emmans Dean, *The Trials of Homeopathy. Origins, Structure and Development* (Essen, 2004), pp. 87ff.
[35] Fangel, Holger J., *Homøopathiske Forsøg ved Sygesengen* (Copenhagen, 1835).
[36] On an answer to this controversy, see Holger J. Fangel, *Svar paa Recensionerne over 'Homøopathiske Forsøg ved Sygesengen'* (Copenhagen, 1835).
[37] Cf. Dean (fn. 34), pp. 106ff.
[38] *Directory 1911/12* (fn. 24), p. 41.
[39] Meyer (fn. 11), p. 125.
[40] *Specielles Illustrirtes Preis-Verzeichniß des Homöopathischen Etablissements von Dr. Willmar Schwabe in Leipzig* (Leipzig, 1887), p. 7.
[41] Alexander Villers, *Internationales Homöopathisches Jahrbuch. Annales homeopathicae.* vol. 2 (Dresden, 1894), p. 31.
[42] *Directory 1911/12* (fn. 24), p. 41.
[43] Volker Jäger, Zur Geschichte der Fa. Willmar Schwabe. In: *MedGG* 10 (1992), pp. 171-188, especially p. 184.
[44] Villers (fn. 41), p. 30.
[45] Donner (fn. 12), p. 237.
[46] Homoeopathy in Denmark. In: *British Journal of Homoeopathy* 13 (1855), p. 694.
[47] *Directory 1911/12* (fn. 24), p. 41.
[48] If not stated otherwise, the following information is according to Winston (fn. 8), p. 569.
[49] Vgl. Carl Bojanus, *Geschichte der Homöopathie in Rußland* (Stuttgart, 1880), pp. 138f., Kotok (fn. 2), p. 32, cf. http://homeoint.org/books4/kotok/1400.htm.
[50] A. Pfaler, Moniaita sanoja Suomen kansan muinaisesta ja nykyisestä lääkitsemis-opista. In: *Duodecim* 4 (1888), pp. 129–139 (http://www.terveysportti.fi/d-htm/articles/1888_7-8_129-139.pdf). For the historical background, cf. Riitta Oittinen, Health, Horror and Dreams for Sale: Patent Medicine and Quackery in Prewar Finland. In: *Historical Aspects of Unconventional Medicine. Approaches, Concepts, Case Studies*, ed. by Robert Jütte, Motzi Eklöf, Marie Nelson (Sheffield, 2001), pp. 119-138.
[51] E. Suolahti, Puoskarintoiminnasta Suomessa. In: *Duodecim* 37 (1921), pp. 246–263.
[52] Significantly, homeopathy is not mentioned in books on the medical history of Finland, see, for instance, Bertel von Bonsdorff, *The History of Medicine in Finland 1828-1918* (Helsinki, 1975).
[53] *Archiv für die homöopathische Heilkunst* 4 (1825), pp. 83f.
[54] See Bojanus (fn. 49), pp. 5f.; Kotok (fn. 2).
[55] G. F. J. Sahmen, *Über die gegenwärtige Stellung der Homöopathie zur bisherigen Heilkunde* (Dorpat, 1825). Cf. http://www.eestiarst.ee/et/export/showpdf.html?id=9.

[56] *Zeitschrift für homöopathische Klinik* 4 (1855), p. 200. Cf. www.eestiarst. ee/et/export/showpdf.html?id=9.
[57] A. C. P. Callissen, *Medizinisches Schriftsteller-Lexicon der Jetzt Lebenden Aerzte, Wundaerzte*, etc., vol. IX, 1832, p. 308.
[58] *AHZ* 26 (1844), Sp. 63 f.
[59] G. O. Kleinert, *Geschichte der Homöopathie* (Leipzig, 1863), p. 165.
[60] Joannes ab Holst, *De structura musculorum* [...] (Dorpat, 1846).
[61] Cf. Meyer (fn. 11), p. 127, Bojanus (fn. 49), p. 44; Callisen (fn. 57), vol. X, p. 277, ibid., vol. XI, p. 24.
[62] Cf. Baur (fn. 32), p. 64.
[63] Bojanus(fn. 49), pp. 79ff.
[64] Alexander Rosendorff, *Neue Erkenntnisse in der Naturheilbehandlung. Aus fünfzigjähriger Praxis* (Bietigheim, 9th ed., 1964), pp. 165f.
[65] On the difficult situation of homeopathy in Russia after World War II, see Kotok, Heresy (fn. 2).
[66] Cf. http://www.lmhint.net/LigaLetter/October98/october98_2.html.
[67] Cf. http://www.lmhint.net/LigaLetter/October01.
[68] Cf. Bojanus (fn. 49), p. 73.
[69] Cf. http://www.homeoint.org/seror/biograph/brutzer.htm.
[70] If not stated otherwise, the following information is according to Marina Afanasieva, The essay on history of homeopathy in Latvia *(http://www.lmhi. net/his_latvia.html)*. The spelling of names in this survey is often faulty and inconsistent. The text has been reprinted by Das (fn. 8), pp. 140-151, omitting, however, all references.
[71] Cf. http://www.lmhint.net/LigaLetter/October99. Cf. Sonja Aevermann, Homöopathie in Lettland. In: *AHZ 249* (2004), pp. 193-194.
[72] Cf. *Zeitschrift für homöopathische Klinik* 14 (1869), p. 14.
[73] Cf. http://www.lmhint.net/LigaLetter/October01.
[74] Donner (fn. 12), p. 266.
[75] *British Homoeopathic Journal* 7 (1849), p. 125.
[76] Meyer (fn. 11), p. 127.
[77] http://www.roots-saknes.lv/Occupations/Doctors/Doctors1862.htm.
[78] Bojanus (fn. 49), p. 123.
[79] Meyer (fn. 11), p. 126.
[80] Villers (fn. 41), p. 40.
[81] *Directory 1911/12* (fn. 24), p. 121.
[82] Donner (fn. 12), p. 266.
[83] Bojanus (fn. 49), p. 145.
[84] Meyer (fn. 11), p. 128. Cf. Janis Kirsis, The Homeopathic Drugstore of Riga. In: *Pharmacy in History 33* (1991), pp. 76-79.
[85] On Petrovsky, see Kotok, Heresy (fn. 2).
[86] Cf. Bojanus (fn. 49), p. 125, p. 128.
[87] http://aconitum.puslapiai.lt/homeopatija/html/english.html.
[88] http://aconitum.puslapiai.lt/homeopatija/html/english.html.
[89] *Zeitschrift für homöopathische Klinik* 21 (1876), p. 111.
[90] *Zeitschrift für homöopathische Klinik* 21 (1876), p. 112.
[91] Cf. Bojanus (fn. 49), p. 135.

[92] Bojanus (fn. 49), p. 123.
[93] Meyer (fn. 11), S 127.
[94] Villers (fn. 41), p. 42.
[95] *Directory 1911/12* (fn. 24), p. 123.
[96] Cf. *Zeitschrift für homöopathische Klinik* 18 (1873), p. 56.
[97] Villers (fn. 41), p. 42.
[98] Villers (fn. 41), p. 40.
[99] Villers (fn. 41), p. 41.
[100] Villers (fn. 41), p. 42.
[101] *Directory 1911/12* (fn. 24), p. 122.
[102] Villers (fn. 41), p. 40.
[103] See Leopold Drexler, Georg Bayr, Die wiedergewonnene Ausstrahlung des früheren Vielvölkerstaates: Österreich. In: Martin Dinges (ed.), *Weltgeschichte der Homöopathie* (Munich, 1996), pp. 74-101, especially: pp. 77f.
[104] Cf. Franz Siegel, *Die Stellung der Homöopathie zur Wissenschaft und zur Oesterreichischen Medizinalverfassung* (Prague, 1859), p. 78; see also Ulrike Gstettner, Gesetzliche Maßnahmen zur Homöopathie in Österreich im 19. Jahrhundert. In: Sonia Horn (ed.), *Homöopathische Spuren. Beiträge zur Geschichte der Homöopathie in Österreich* (Vienna, 2003), pp. 93-106, especially p. 101.
[105] Ignaz Rudolph Bischoff, *Ansichten über das bisherige Heilverfahren und über die ersten Grundsätze der homöopathischen Krankheitslehre* (Prague, 1819), preface (no pagination).
[106] Samuel Hahnemann, *Organon racionální léčby*; z nřmčiny přeložila Emílie Harantová ; předmluva Jiří Čehovský (Prague, 1993).
[107] James Tyler Kent, *Repertorium homeopatické Materie mediky*, z angličtiny přeložil Luděk Ryba (Prague, 1994). The same applies to materia medica books by Boericke and Pulford as well as to Allen's *Keynotes;* cf. Winston (fn. 8), p. 568.
[108] 11th Congress (fn. 30), p. 80.
[109] *Zeitschrift des Vereins der homöopathischen Ärzte Oesterreichs* 2 (1857), pp. 186f.
[110] *Zeitschrift des Vereins der homöopathischen Ärzte Oesterreichs* 1 (1857), p. 411.
[111] http://www.lmhint.net/LigaLetter/October01.
[112] Cf. *Österreichisches Biographisches Lexikon*, vol. 6, pp. 77/78; Hannelore Petry, *Die Wiener Homöopathie* 1842-1848 (medical dissertation University of Mainz, 1954), p. 315.
[113] See the obituary in *Prager Medicinische Monatsschrift [...] (PMM)* 1 (1853), pp. 109ff.
[114] Cf. Elias Altschul, Materialien zur Geschichte der Homöopathie in Böhmen und Mähren, in: *PMM* 5 (1856), pp. 145-151, especially p. 147. On Schaller, see Auguste Rapou, *Histoire de la doctrine Homeopathique. Son état actuel dans les principales contrées de l'Europe*, vol. 2 (Paris, London, 1847), pp. 3ff.
[115] See the obituary in *PMM* 5 (1857), pp. 77f.
[116] Cf. *PMM* 5 (1857), pp. 81-83.
[117] Cf. [firstname unknown] Hože, Materialien zur Geschichte der Homöopathie in Mähren. In: *PMM* 4 (1856), pp. 177-185, especially p. 179.
[118] Cf. Kleinert (fn. 59), p. 323.

[119] Cf. Hože (fn. 117), p. 178.
[120] Cf. Joseph Attomyr, *Briefe über die Homöopathie*, vol. 2 (Leipzig, 1833), pp. 63f.
[121] Cf. Hože (fn. 117), pp. 181f.
[122] The letter to Dr Löwe in Prague is reprinted in *PMM* 5 (1857), p. 32.
[123] Cf. Attomyr (fn. 120), vol. 2, pp. 63f.
[124] Cf. the letter of thanks by Dieble, quoted by J. Rutherfurd Russell, *History and Heroes of the Art of Medicine* (London, 1861), p. 426. Cf. also Josef Buchner, *Resultate der Kranken-Behandlung allopathischer und homöopathischer Schule* (Munich, 1848), p. 6.
[125] Meyer (fn. 11), pp. 32ff.
[126] *Zeitschrift für homöopathische Klinik* 9 (1864), p. 135.
[127] Villers (fn. 41), pp. 26ff.
[128] Cf. Christian Lucae, *Homöopathie an deutschsprachigen Universitäten. Die Bestrebungen zu ihrer Institutionalisierung von 1812 bis 1945* (Heidelberg, 1998), pp. 63ff.
[129] Josef Adamec (ed.), *Biografický slovník Pražské Lékarské Fakulty: 1348-1939 [Biographical Dictionary of the Medical Faculty in Prague, 1348-1939]* (Prague, 1988), p. 74. Cf. Eduard Huber, Geschichte der Homöopathie in Österreich (Cisleithanien). In: Carl Heinigke (ed.), *Sammlungen wissenschaftlicher Abhandlungen auf dem Gebiet der Homöopathie*, serie 1, no. 2 (Leipzig, 1878), pp. 43-56, especially p. 54.
[130] *Neue Zeitschrift für homöopathische Klinik* 5 (1860), pp. 33f.
[131] *Zeitschrift für homöopathische Klinik* 10 (1865), pp. 127f.
[132] Cf. Adamec (fn. 129), p. 113.
[133] Cf. *11th Congress* (fn. 30), p. 80.
[134] *11th Congress* (fn. 30), p. 80.
[135] I thank Dr Gerhard Peithner (Vienna) for this information.
[136] Winston (fn. 8), p. 568.
[137] *British Journal of Homoeopathy* 8 (1850), pp. 279f.
[138] Meyer (fn. 11), p. 78.
[139] *British Journal of Homoeopathy* 8 (1850), p. 278.
[140] Cf.. Huber (fn. 129), p. 55.
[141] Cf. Huber (fn. 129), p. 56.
[142] Cf. Kleinert (fn. 59), p. 322.
[143] Altschul, Materialien (fn. 114), p. 148.
[144] Siegel (fn. 104), p. 50.
[145] *PMM* 5 (1857), p. 152, cf. *PMM* 6 (1858), pp. 75ff.
[146] Cf. Gstettner (fn. 104), pp. 104ff.
[147] Rapou (fn. 114), vol. 2, pp. 37f.
[148] *Neue Zeitschrift für homöopathische Klinik* 5 (1860), Nr. 14.
[149] Villers (fn. 41), p. 27.
[150] *11th Congress* (fn. 30), p. 80.
[151] Jäger (fn. 43), p. 184.
[152] *11th Congress* (fn. 30), p. 80.
[153] *PMM* 6 (1858), pp. 37f.; pp. 54f.; Bd. 9 (1861), pp. 28f.
[154] *PMM* 10 (1862), pp. 152ff.

[155] Cf. Altschul, Materialien (fn. 114), p. 150.
[156] Cf. Attomyr (fn. 120).
[157] http://www.lmhint.net/LigaLetter/October98/october98_2.html.
[158] *Zeitschrift des Vereins der homöopathischen Ärzte Oesterreichs* 1 (1862), pp. 190f.
[159] Kócián/Kölnei, Geschichte (fn. 5), p. 216.
[160] http://www.lmhint.net/LigaLetter/October98/october98_2.html
[161] http://www.homeo.sk/fanklub/ktosme.asp
[162] Cf. *AHZ* 52 (1856), pp. 33-36; *AHZ* 178 (1930), pp. 124-126.
[163] Attomyr (fn. 120), vol. 1, p. 26.
[164] Attomyr (fn. 120), vol. 1, p. 141.
[165] Rapou (fn. 114), vol. 1, p. 400. Cf. Melitta Schmideberg, Die Geschichte der homöopathischen Bewegung in Ungarn. In: *AHZ* 178 (1930), pp. 87-134, 210-250, especially p. 224.
[166] Villers (fn. 41), p. 27; *Directory 1911/12* (fn. 23), p. 36.
[167] http://www.lmhint.net/LigaLetter/October98/october98_2.html.
[168] Villers (fn. 41), p. 27.
[169] http://www.lmhint.net/LigaLetter/March99.
[170] Carl Heinrich Rosenberg, *Fortschritte und Leistungen der Homöopathie in und außer Ungarn* (Leipzig, 1843), p. 60.
[171] Cf. Baur (fn. 30), pp. 53f.; Laszlo Kiss, Ki volt Hahnemann Organon-jának elsö „magyarítója"? In: *Orvosi Hetilap* 131 (1990), S. 2552-2555.
[172] Cf. Schmideberg (fn. 165), p. 113.
[173] I owe these bibliographical details to the study by Kócián/Kölnei, Geschichte (fn. 5), p. 206.
[174] *Zeitschrift für homöopathische Klinik* 11 (1866), p. 23.
[175] Schmideberg (fn. 165), p. 110.
[176] Cf. László Kiss, A magyarországi homeopatákelsö egyesülete (1843-1845?). The First Society of Hungarian Homeopaths (1843-1845). In: *Orvostörténeti Közlemények (Communicationes de historia artis medicinae)* 190-193 (2005), pp. 223-228. This study which is based on archival research contradicts the information provided by Schmideberg (fn. 165), p. 92, Kócián/Kölnei, Geschichte (fn. 5), pp. 211f.
[177] Cf. the constitution, reprinted in: *Zeitschrift für homöopathische Klinik* 9 (1864), pp. 71f.
[178] Koltay (fn. 5), p. 61.
[179] http://www.lmhint.net/LigaLetter/October01/.
[180] Rosenberg (fn. 170), pp. 74f.
[181] Meyer (fn. 11).
[182] Tihamér von Balogh, Statistik der Homöopathie in Ungarn, in: *AHZ* 84 (1872), pp. 119-120, 143-144, 168, 176, 183-184, especially p. 120.
[183] Villers (fn. 41), pp. 26ff.
[184] *Directory 1911/12* (fn. 24), pp. 35ff.
[185] Winston (fn. 8), p. 571.
[186] *Sitzungsberichte des X. Kongresses* (fn. 25), p. 470.
[187] Cf. Kócián/Kölnei, Geschichte (fn. 5), pp. 204ff.

[188] Schmideberg (fn. 165), p. 90.
[189] Schmideberg (fn. 165), p. 90.
[190] Cf. Rosenberg (fn. 170), pp. 92ff., Schmideberg (fn. 165), p. 89.
[191] Kócián/Kölnei, Geschichte (fn. 5), p. 213.
[192] Schmideberg (fn. 165), p. 105.
[193] *Zeitschrift für homöopathische Klinik* 17 (1872), p. 16. Cf. Kócián/Kölnei, Geschichte (fn. 5), p. 212.
[194] Schmideberg (fn. 165), p. 102.
[195] Balogh (fn. 182), p. 120.
[196] *Zeitschrift für homöopathische Klinik* 21 (1876), pp. 21f.
[197] Schmideberg (fn. 165), p. 103.
[198] *11th Congress* (fn. 30), p. 63. Cf. Schmideberg (fn. 165), p. 112, Kócián/Kölnei, Schimert (fn. 5), pp. 101-106.
[199] Schmideberg (fn. 165), p. 91.
[200] Cf. Balogh (fn. 182), p. 168.
[201] See Lucae (fn. 128), pp. 73f., Kócián/Kölnei,Geschichte (fn. 5), pp. 213f.
[202] period of rapid economic growth in Germany, Austria and Hungary after 1871 (translator's note)
[203] *11th Congress* (fn. 30), p. 63.
[204] *Sitzungsberichte des X. Kongresses* (fn. 25), p. 470.
[205] See Balogh (fn. 182), p. 176.
[206] http://www.lmhint.net/LigaLetter/October01/.
[207] The law is quoted by Schmideberg (fn. 165), p. 102.
[208] Bernstein [Karl Hugo], *Mosaik* (Leipzig, 1837), p . 129.
[209] Bernstein (fn. 208), p. 298.
[210] Meyer (fn. 11), p. 76.
[211] *Sitzungsberichte des X. Kongresses* (fn. 25), p. 470.
[212] Cf. Schmideberg (fn. 165), p. 88.
[213] Cf. Rosenberg (fn. 170), pp. 55ff.
[214] http://www.lmhint.net/LigaLetter/October98/october98_2.html. See also Winston (fn. 8), p. 571.
[215] *Zeitschrift für homöopathische Klinik* 20 (1875), p. 52. A sickness fund named "Zion" is mentioned there.
[216] *Zeitschrift des Vereins der homöopathischen Ärzte Oesterreichs* 1 (1857), p. 300.
[217] Kócián/Kölnei, Geschichte (fn. 5), p. 212.
[218] *Bibliotheca Homeopathica. International bibliography of homeopathic literature*, compiled by J. Baur, K.-H. Gypser, G. von Keller, P.W. Thomas (Gouda, 1984), p. 75
[219] Rosenberg (fn. 170), p. 140. For his biography, see Daniel Bertsch, *Anton Prokesch von Osten (1795-1876). Ein Diplomat Österreichs in Athen und an der Hohen Pforte. Beiträge zur Wahrnehmung des Orients im Europa des 19. Jahrhunderts* (Munich, 2005).
[220] According to the editor A. N. Goudas in: *I Iatriki Melissa* [the medical honey bee] 6 (1858/59). For this and other information on Greece I thank Dr M. Ruisinger (Erlangen).

[221] Friedrich Zuccarini: Pest, Cholera und Aerzte in Konstantinopel. In: *Das Ausland* 4 (1831), pp. 1203; 1211f., especially p. 1211.
[222] Rosenberg (fn. 170), p. 140.
[223] *British Journal of Homoeopathy* 9 (1851), p. 506.
[224] *Directory 1911/12* (fn. 24), p. 133.
[225] I thank the former Greek ambassador Anthony Nomikos (Athens) for this information. Cf. Winston (fn. 8), p. 571.
[226] http://www.homeopathy.gr/HHMS.html.
[227] http://www.lmhint.net/LigaLetter/October98/october98_2.html.
[228] *World Directory of the Homeopathic Physicians* (Marseille, 1973), no pagination.
[229] http://www.wholehealthnow.com/homeopathy_pro/greece.html.
[230] Cf. Das (fn. 8), p. 91.
[231] http://www.lmhing.net/LigaLetter/October98/october98_2.html.
[231] Cf. *Griechenland-Zeitung* (9th December 2005), p.14.